IS TH............CHILDBIRTH?

ABOUT THE AUTHOR

Juliet Rix is a freelance journalist. After taking a degree in biological sciences and history of art at Cambridge University, she joined the BBC, working in television and radio. She spent a couple of years as a foreign correspondent in Indonesia before returning to the UK to have her first child. She lives in London with her husband and two young sons.

IS THERE SEX AFTER CHILDBIRTH?

*A couple's guide to survival through pregnancy,
birth and parenthood*

JULIET RIX

Thorsons
An Imprint of HarperCollinsPublishers

For Rod and our two sons

Thorsons
An Imprint of HarperCollins*Publishers*
77–85 Fulham Palace Road,
Hammersmith, London W6 8JB
1160 Battery Street,
San Francisco, California 94111–1213

Published by Thorsons 1995

10 9 8 7 6 5 4 3 2 1

© Juliet Rix 1995

Juliet Rix asserts the moral right to
be identified as the author of this work

A catalogue record for this book
is available from the British Library

ISBN 0 7225 2957 0

Printed in Great Britain
by HarperCollinsManufacturing Glasgow

CONTENTS

ACKNOWLEDGEMENTS

First I would like to thank those of my friends who talked openly about this normally taboo subject after our first children were born and so alerted me to the need for this book. And then the many others who have since shared their experiences in writing or over the phone specifically for this book.

I am extremely grateful to the many experts who talked to me or read part or all of the manuscript. Gynaecologist and sex therapist Fran Reader and research midwife Rona McCandlish of the National Perinatal Epidemiology Unit (NPEU) were both exceptionally generous with their time and knowledge, as were others at the NPEU, especially Mary Renfrew and Adrian Grant. At Relate (the old marriage guidance council) Jane Hawksley, Angela Martin and Zelda West-Meads were all very helpful, as were Christopher Clulow, director of the Tavistock Institute of Marital Studies, and Penny Mansfield at One Plus One. I am very grateful to the NCT and many of the individuals within it, to Toni Bellfield at the FPA, to Beth Alder and Jerri Thoman, to Mr Peter Greenhouse and Dr Patricia Munday, and to obstetricians John Spencer and Margaret Hobbiss. Many thanks must also go to the authors of A Guide to Effective Care in Pregnancy and Childbirth, Murray Enkin, Marc J. N. C. Keirse and Iain Chalmers.

I donot know what I would have done without Claire Lowe at the British Medical Association library and her help in tracking down medical papers; the staff at the Royal College of Midwives Library were also always patient and helpful. The NCT, Guardian Women and the Daily Telegraph health page all helped me to find people to talk about this subject, as did my own antenatal teacher Yvonne Moore, who also supported me through a second pregnancy that was over-busy partly due to the writing of this book.

I would like to thank my agent Jane Conway-Gordon and my editor Sarah Sutton for believing in the book and for their understanding when pregnancy and the birth of my second son slowed progress for a while.

Last, but by no means least, my heartfelt thanks go to my husband, Rod, for backing the idea of the book, commenting on the manuscript and putting up with late evenings spent at the keyboard when they should have been spent with him!

INTRODUCTION

When I was first working on this book I told several people I was writing aboout sex in pregnancy and after childbirth. The parents among them usually gave a slightly embarassed laugh and said, 'That will be a short book.' In fact, of course, sex itself is only a part of the book, just as it is only a part of your relationship. The state of your sex life affects the state of your relationship and vice versa. And ultimately it is not the sex that really matters, but you. Whether and how you have sex is not in itself important, but the relationship is important, both to you and to your children.

Pregnancy, birth and early parenthood are times of intense experience and change. Relationships have a lot of adapting to do. This is perhaps even more true now than ever before; the shape of marriage and cohabitation today is not built around the arrival of children in the way that it used to be, and the current generation of new parents have also grown up with the idea that we should be better at talking about sex, and perhaps even at doing it, than our predecessors.

Pregnancy, birth and early parenthood unquestionably affect most couples' sex lives, and yet this is rarely talked about. The plentiful discussion of sex and copious books on the subject rarely address the issues of sex and parenthood. As children of the 'permissive society', today's new parents may assume that if it isn't talked about them they are the only ones having problems. In fact, this just seems to be one of the last taboos.

Relationship counsellors and sex therapists say they often find that even when they do not see a couple until years later, problems frequently date back to the birth of the first child. One sex therapist added that she has seen a number of couples in the months after the birth who think they have a sexual problem when in fact they are normal new parents in the first postnatal year!

This book was conceived (as it were) when I told a male friend and father of a nine-month-old that research had found over 50 per cent of couples had not returned to pre-pregnancy levels of sexual activity a year after the birth. There was an audible sigh of relief. Then he said, 'Yesterday I was embarassed about our sex life. I thought there was something wrong with us. Now I know it is normal.'

This one fact made all the difference to him, and I felt sad and angry that he should have gone through all that extra worry for lack of a bit of basic information.

I give more space in the book to that period after birth than to pregnancy because afterwards seems to be the time when otherwise happy relationships suffer most. Pregnancy is so obviously not a 'normal' time and you can put up with most things if you know they will last no more than nine months. After birth there is a (mistaken) tendency to assume things will get straight back to 'norma;' and a feeling that if they don't they never will. This isn't true of course. Early parenthood is almost as temporary as pregnancy, though it may not feel that way!

The fact is that a couple's relationship – sexual and otherwise – does not generally get the same time or attention after a baby as it did before. But this does not have to be a problem. This book hopes to offer a layman's look at what is known in this area, a sense of what is normal, and some ideas on coping with any problems (physical or emotional) that do arise.

The book is aimed at couples. It is intended to be read by both of you. When I say 'you' in the text it usually means you as a couple, reading it. Inevitably the pregnancy section talks to and about women more than men, but otherwise only rarely does 'you' refer to one or other partner.

I use the word 'partner', for all its inadequacies, simply because I could find no better alternative to cover parents with and without a marriage certificate. For the baby I have used 'he' and 'she' (and occasionally it) at random.

Dividing up the information in a book like this is inevitably somewhat arbitrary, so if you cannot find some information where you would expect it, do have a look in the Index in case it is somewhere else. Some parts of the book may not seem directly relevant to sex, but getting a birth you are happy with and a home life that does not create resentment are vital to your sexual – and general – happiness.

Take from the book what is useful to you and forget the rest. If it gives a few people a few useful ideas, and opens up the subject for discussion, I will feel justified in having written it.

And a word of reassurance: It is not all doom and gloom for your sex life. Many parents I spoke to said that once through the postnatal period of adjustment, their sex lives were actually better. They summarized it as 'quantity down, quality up!'.

PART ONE

SEX IN PREGNANCY

It should come as no surprise that pregnancy is likely to affect your sex life. It may, however, come as a surprise just how much you are affected and in what way. Research studies have found two main patterns of sexual activity during pregnancy. Either there is a reduction in the frequency of love-making, with a steady decline as the pregnancy progresses, or love-making dips in the first trimester, increases in the second and falls off again in the third.

These are, however, only statistical patterns. Individual couples experience almost every variation, from no sex at all to the most rampant sexual activity of their lives, or any mixture of the two.

I was more interested in sex right up to the last couple of months. We had sex more often until seven months, and then less.

We both went off sex and did it a lot less often.

We had sex about twice when I first got pregnant, then I just didn't feel like it. Towards the very end I got completely randy. From about seven months I was rampant...I felt like ringing my partner up at work and saying 'come home quick.' I began to understand the jokes about the milkman!

Sex was great, and the same as before my pregnancy until exactly 30 weeks. Then my libido switched off totally.

Sex in pregnancy was never a problem for me. In some ways

it was better. I really felt like a woman when I was pregnant. I really enjoyed sex. The problems came afterwards.

Our sex life was about the same as before pregnancy.

I felt ill in the first trimester and worried about the baby in the last, but in between our sex life improved. Sex drive and pleasure increased.

No big changes in [our] sex life except I felt very sick in the first trimester so [I was] not much interested in sex in those months.

When expecting my first child I didn't want to know about sex – even the word made me retch. But when expecting my second I was practically swinging from the chandelier (if we had had one).

There are many reasons for the patterns of sexual activity and desire in pregnancy; physical, psychological and medical. What you want and what you do may be quite different, as for example when sex is abandoned on medical advice. Frequency also does not necessarily link to either desire or satisfaction. Some pregnant women get great pleasure out of sex but just can't find the energy to do it very often. Others have plenty of desire but are too worried about the baby to actually do it. Men may also worry about the baby, and some men find their sexual feelings for their partner considerably affected by the changes pregnancy brings.

What follows is a trimester-by-trimester guide to the possible effects of pregnancy on your sex life. Trimesters in this context are really just a rough split of pregnancy into three stages – not necessarily of exactly three months each. Don't be surprised if your 'first trimester' lasts four months or your last only two months. Some people hardly notice three parts to their pregnancy at all. Also, even if you are already part-way through your pregnancy, do read the chapters on the earlier trimester(s) as information that these contain also applies to the later stages of pregnancy.

1

THE FIRST TRIMESTER

The Physical Effects

Some women sail through the first few months of pregnancy barely aware they are pregnant. Many others, however, have a variety of symptoms that can be anything from slightly to very disruptive of day-to-day life and sex.

The first physical effects of pregnancy sometimes start before you can even confirm you are pregnant. 'Morning sickness' (which can happen at any time of day) or extreme fatigue may set in almost from the start. These may be swiftly followed by enlarged and tender breasts and a need to urinate frequently – none of which is very conducive to nights (or days) of passion.

In the first trimesters [of all my pregnancies] I felt sick, bloated, chronically tired and generally unwell – sex life plummeted.

Laura, daughter 8 yrs, sons 5 yrs and 18 m

In the first trimester my breasts became *very* tender and painful to the touch. I felt like biting my partner or hitting him over the head when he tried to make love to me. Instead of telling him this, I lay there and gritted my teeth. This was not a good idea, as I subsequently came to realize.

Katie, son 2 yrs

The early months are also the time when the pregnancy is least obvious. No concessions will be made at work, on public transport, or even amongst friends if you have not yet made your pregnancy public. After the first week or two even partners may tend to forget that this woman who looks the same as ever is in fact working for two and may be feeling exhausted and unwell.

> I was so desperately tired I could not believe everything was all right. I got as far as the obstetrician before I was reassured. I went down with a bug and took ages to shake it off and I kept almost fainting if I stood for more than about 10 minutes. My partner was delighted about the pregnancy and very loving. He wanted to show it by making love. I simply couldn't face it.
>
> **Jennifer, son 2 yrs**

If you do get around to making love, you may already find physical changes or differences in your sexual needs. (*See also The Emotional Effects, page 11.*) Breasts may have to be left out of the proceedings because they hurt, or they may be a focus of attention because they are for the first time large and firm – or, frustratingly, they may be both a focus of attention and out of bounds! Some men and women find that even if the breasts are not tender they seem so obviously preparing for another job (i.e. breastfeeding) that it is difficult to enjoy them sexually.

The genital area may also be changing.

> I found that it was very uncomfortable if my partner penetrated fully. It was as if the cervix was lower and he was bumping into it. In our first pregnancy this was part of the reason we had very little sex. Second time around we were just careful about how far he went in, or did other things.
>
> **Natasha, son 3 yrs**

The best way to deal with these changes is to talk openly and honestly to each other. Not all couples find it easy to discuss sex or express their needs and preferences. In fact, many find it very difficult. Some lose their inhibitions after going through labour, birth and early parenthood together. But this does not help you much first time around. If you are not already good at talking about what works for you sexually, this is a very good time to start. Learning to work around sore breasts or changed needs at this stage is extremely useful, as the changes are only likely to get more acute and if you continue to make love, there will be more to work around as the pregnancy progresses – not to mention after the birth.

For those whose sex drive remains intact and for whom there is no medical reason not to make love, pregnancy can be a time for discovering new ways of giving and receiving pleasure. Not wanting to, or not being able to do what you normally do can be quite liberating if you allow yourselves the sexual openness to explore alternatives.

'Alternatives' does not have to mean sexual acrobatics. What is an 'alternative' depends on what you already do. Some couples are obviously more adventurous than others. If you need a few ideas, take a look at Appendix B.

Try to keep an open mind. There is a lot of misplaced guilt around when it comes to sex, and trying new positions often brings it to the fore. If you enjoy what you are doing and it isn't hurting anyone, then it is hard to see what is wrong with it. It is obviously vital, however, to be true to yourselves. Do not push or feel pushed into anything you don't BOTH feel comfortable with.

Pain or Discomfort During Sex

When you are not pregnant, sexual excitement leads to a rising of the uterus and lengthening and ballooning of the vagina. The way this happens also means that the penis tends to prod behind the cervix rather than on to the cervix itself. Sometimes in pregnancy this movement does not happen and you can feel pain or discomfort from the penis bumping against the cervix. Early in pregnancy this is probably due to hormonal changes. Later it may happen because of the weight of the pregnant uterus. This is nothing to worry about, but it is best to avoid knocking the cervix too hard.

In early pregnancy it is also occasionally possible for the prodding penis to trap an ovary between the back of the cervix and the sacrum (the tail bone), causing pain during intercourse. At the beginning of pregnancy, the ovary that released the now-fertilized egg is usually enlarged with a small cyst on it producing a hormone to maintain the pregnancy until the placenta is ready to take over at about four months. Once the placenta is fully functioning the ovary shrinks back to normal.

Hormonal changes also soften the ligaments that hold your bones in place. This is to allow greater opening of the pelvis for the birth, but in the mean time it can cause the bones at the front and back of the pelvis to shift slightly in relation to each other. The positions adopted for intercourse may place added strain on the pelvis and can occasionally cause pain during sex. Changing positions may help.

If you have discomfort from the surface of the vulva or vagina, or a feeling of being too dry, this may be due to thrush or some other infection (see below) or to a simple lack of lubrication. Dryness without any infection is most likely to be due to not being sufficiently aroused – because of tension, worry, being unable to relax – or simply being too tired (see Chapter 8). In this case you can use a bit of extra lubrication like KY Jelly (or any water-based lubricant), or even spit. But do not use these methods to replace proper arousal or to mask fears or worries. Talk your concerns through together and try to be open both about the pregnancy and about your sexual needs.

Is Sex Safe?

Many parents-to-be get very concerned about the safety of sex in pregnancy, and whether in the early months it might cause miscarriage. Research so far suggests that sex is safe in an uncomplicated pregnancy and it is now regarded as inappropriate for health professionals to advise couples against making love unless there is a specific reason. In uncomplicated pregnancies the possibility of causing stress and tension in the relationship by banning sex is now thought to outweigh any potential benefit.

Most early miscarriages are due to an embryo that has something wrong with it and is never going to develop properly. Other causes include problems with the mother's immune system, abnormal uterus, incompetent (weak) cervix, hormone deficiencies, and some illnesses. Miscarriages do of course sometimes happen shortly after making love, but this does not mean it would not have happened had you not made love. Gynaecologist and sex therapist Fran Reader says, 'Sex might sometimes be the trigger that makes you miscarry at that particular moment but it is not the cause.'

Saying that sex is safe in normal pregnancy does, however, assume that couples will listen to the woman's body. The research that suggests that sex is not harmful did not compare couples told to have sex with couples told not to, but those who chose to and those who chose not to. It may be that some of the substantial minority who chose not to have sex at certain stages of the pregnancy (including the first trimester) were right. People often know much more about their bodies than medical science can explain, and it may be that women's bodies 'know' when sex is OK and when it is not. If a woman feels strongly that sex is not a good idea, or finds any aspect of sex uncomfortable, her feelings should be taken seriously.

Complications That May Mean No Sex

PREVIOUS MISCARRIAGE

If you have had an early miscarriage in a previous pregnancy, some doctors and midwives will advise against having sex in the first trimester or will suggest that you abstain at those times when the first few periods would have been due. This is an 'on the safe side' policy. There is no clear evidence that it makes any difference, but nor is there proof positive that it does not.

BLEEDING

Spotting (very small amounts of blood) or more copious bleeding is not uncommon in the first trimester and often leads to no further problems. It is, however, known medically as 'threatened miscarriage' and will be treated as such until proved otherwise. The quantities of blood involved in spotting mean that it is unlikely to be due to a serious problem. The more blood, the more worrying, but even a patch or small pool of blood is by no means certain to signal the end of the pregnancy. Most doctors and midwives would advise abstaining from sex until you know that the bleeding is nothing serious, although once again this is an 'on the safe side' policy rather than one based on known facts.

If the bleeding happens straight after making love, the blood may be coming from the cervix rather than the uterus. Occasionally part of the lining of the cervical canal is visible on the surface of the cervix. This is (rather misleadingly) called a cervical erosion. The lining of the canal is thinner than the usual surface of the cervix, so it is more likely to bleed when it is bumped during intercourse.

There is no danger to the pregnancy but the bleeding may happen repeatedly during or after intercourse unless you are careful that penetration is not too deep or thrusting too vigorous. It is difficult ever to be 100 per cent certain that this minor 'cervical erosion' is the cause of bleeding, so it is probably best to try and prevent further bleeds if you do not want to go through repeated periods of worry or medical investigation.

A rarer cause of non-uterine bleeding is a polyp. Polyps are small grape-like lumps rich in blood vessels that grow from the lining of the uterus or cervical canal. They pose no threat to the pregnancy.

If the blood is thought to be coming from the uterus – or the doctor or midwife simply cannot tell – you may be offered a scan to check that everything is OK. If the scan is normal and bleeding has stopped, there is no medical reason why you should not return to making love as usual. If you are in doubt or either of you would feel more comfortable abstaining until the end of the first trimester, then go with your gut feeling.

Sometimes copious bleeding is due to a twin pregnancy in which one of the two foetuses has been lost. Once this is established and the second embryo is shown to be OK, you can go back to normal love-making.

If at any time you pass anything other than plain blood from the vagina (such as blood clots or other material), it is probably worth keeping it to show your doctor as it may give a clue as to the cause of the bleeding.

PAIN

Painful abdominal cramps can also be a sign of impending miscarriage, although again not necessarily. It is probably wise to abstain from sex until the cause of the pain is established, especially if the cramping comes during or after love-making.

See also Chapters 2 and 3.

If at any time you are advised by your doctor or midwife not to have sex, do make sure you know exactly what is meant. Often couples get out of the consulting room and realize that they don't really know what is not allowed or why. This can lead to stressful attempts to avoid all sexual activity, or to worry and guilt if it is not avoided. If you are in any doubt, ask: Is it penetration that is to be avoided? deep penetration? orgasm? semen in the vagina? or sexual arousal? And for how long do you need to abstain – throughout pregnancy? until 12 weeks, 14 weeks? 37 weeks? Although it may be easier said than done, try to ask straight questions and insist on straight answers.

Infections

Some genital or sexually transmitted diseases (STDs) can be a particular problem in pregnancy – either because pregnancy makes a woman more prone to them or because they can damage her and/or the baby. If at any time during pregnancy you notice an abnormal genital discharge (for women: a different colour, smelly, pus-like; for men: any discharge at all), soreness, itching, a rash on the genitals, or pain when urinating, it is worth investigating.

There are two simple precautions you can take to reduce the likelihood of infection: If you include the anus in any of your sexual activity, be sure that anything that has touched the anus (even a finger) does not then go into the vagina before being thoroughly washed. And do not have casual sexual partners or have sex with someone who does – or, if you do, use a condom. However careful you are, you can still get an infection. Two of the most common, thrush and Bacterial Vaginosis, generally are not sexually transmitted and often appear apparently spontaneously (*see below*).

If either of you has ever had a 'high-risk' lifestyle (multiple sexual partners, homosexual partners, intravenous drug use, unprotected sex in high-risk parts of the world) – even some years ago –

you could be carrying an STD of which you are unaware. It might be worth asking for an extra test at your antenatal clinic, GP's surgery or at a GU clinic (Genito-Urinary Medicine clinic, STD clinic, Sexual Health clinic). At these special clinics you can both be checked at the same time, there are experts in the field, and confidentiality is guaranteed by law.

Most STDs can be carried for years by either sex without any symptoms. Sometimes – particularly with Herpes and genital warts – a woman may have her first visible attack during pregnancy even though she is not newly infected.

It is important to remember that a new diagnosis does not mean a new disease, since this also means that there has not necessarily been any recent sexual disloyalty in your relationship, or indeed any disloyalty at all. One of you may have contracted the infection before the two of you even met. For more on STDs in pregnancy, see Appendix C. There follows a little more on the two most common genital complaints in pregnancy.

Thrush
(also known as Candida Albicans or Monilia)

This is extremely common generally, and even more common in pregnancy. It is also often harder to get rid of when you are pregnant. Thrush can cause anything from no symptoms to extreme itching, soreness and discharge. It is not in the least dangerous to either the woman or the baby, but untreated it can be a considerable nuisance to both.

You can try 'home' remedies like live yoghurt (wiped around the vagina and vulva) or tea-tree oil pessaries or cream. Tea-tree oil is a natural anti-fungal and anti-bacterial available from some chemists and health food shops. Even if these treatments have worked for you in the past they may not be strong enough in pregnancy. Of the common conventional treatments, clotrimazole (*Canestan*) has been shown to be more effective than *Nystatin* for pregnant women. Both are regarded as safe in pregnancy.

If the thrush is not bothering you too much or if it keeps recurring after treatment you can delay further treatment until shortly before the due date. It is worth doing a course of treatment then, otherwise the baby may pick up the infection during the birth and develop oral thrush (white patches in the mouth). Oral thrush is not dangerous but it can be a real nuisance and should be treated (with over-the-counter *Daktarin* gel or prescription *Nystan*). Any thrush remaining in the vagina after the birth should be easily cleared up. You are no longer pregnant and no longer especially susceptible.

If you do decide to 'live with' the thrush for a while, your (male) partner may want to be vigilant about washing under the foreskin so that you do not ping-pong the infection back and forth between you. If he should get thrush, he may be able to get rid of it with careful washing under the foreskin with water and no soap, yoghurt or tea-tree oil cream. Otherwise, *Canestan* cream will do the job.

Bacterial Vaginosis (BV)
(also known as Gardnerella, anaerobic vaginosis or anaerobes)

This is also very common, with perhaps a third of women getting it at some time in their lives. It may produce anything from no obvious symptoms to a watery white-to-greyish discharge with a fishy smell and perhaps soreness. It is not sexually transmitted and will not be passed to the male partner.

Standard treatment for BV is the antibiotic metranidazole (*Flagyl*). *Flagyl* is not generally given in the first trimester of pregnancy in the UK or at any stage in pregnancy in the US, although the evidence that it is harmful is uncertain. A cream, *Dalacin*, has recently become available. It is used directly into the vagina and is therefore thought to be safer. *Flagyl* should also not be taken while breastfeeding, as it can sour the milk.

BV is not much of a problem in itself, but it is now thought that if it is present during the third trimester it may be associated with an increased risk of premature labour. More research is currently in progress.

The Emotional Effects

The knowledge that you are pregnant can bring anything from a surge of happiness and love to total panic, or possibly both.

Confirmation of a planned and wanted pregnancy often brings extra tenderness to a relationship. Pregnancy can be a very warm time between you, and particularly in the first flush of excitement you may find renewed affection for each other. Men may feel protective and loving. But don't expect this necessarily to mean a great sex life. For all the reasons mentioned above and below, sex is often not at the top of the agenda in the first 12–14 weeks of pregnancy.

If the pregnancy is unwanted or unexpected it can bring considerable tensions. One or both of you may feel trapped – in a relationship that has not yet settled, or simply by the responsibility for which you do not feel ready.

> The pregnancy was unplanned but welcome...We had only been together a few months. It all happened very, very quickly. Part of me was convinced this was absolutely the right thing to do. The other half was kicking against it like nobody's business. I panicked because of these enormous threats to my independence. In the first three months I was sick quite a lot and I went right off Lawrence. By three months we were going to family therapy. We split up and I spent a couple of weeks facing up to what it would be like (on my own). We got back together, talked a lot and finally took the plunge and got married...From then on we were fine, and from seven months our sex life was brilliant right up until about three days before the baby was born.
>
> Nicola, son 10 m

Needless to say, these difficulties are made even worse if one of you wanted a baby and the other did not, or if there was any difference of opinion about what to do when the pregnancy was confirmed. This of course leaves even greater room for resentment and (often unreasonable) allocation of blame.

Even a wanted pregnancy may bring tensions. Fears about loss of independence are not limited to those with shock pregnancies. Women, and occasionally men, worry about their ability to be a good parent. Men, and occasionally women, worry about providing for the new family and may feel trapped in a job they do not particularly like. Women often have at least moments of resenting the fact that all the physical changes fall on them, while men may feel left out of the process.

In pregnancy, women often become more emotionally dependent. They may suddenly feel terribly vulnerable, and their emotions go up and down like a yo-yo. Some couples enjoy a new interdependence, but for others it can be quite a shock, leaving the woman wondering where her strength has gone and the man feeling leant on and claustrophobic.

Any tension in your relationship can affect your sex life, but negative feelings relating to pregnancy are even more likely to do so. Pregnancy is, after all, the direct result of sex. Many couples nowadays do not really link sex and reproduction until they try to conceive or become pregnant. Pregnancy brings you face to face with the fundamental purpose of sex. If a pregnancy is wanted this can be very exciting. If it is not, or if you are feeling ambivalent, it can be off-putting.

All these issues need to be recognized if they arise. Try to talk in a blame-free way, and start to understand how the other is feeling. It is a recurring theme of this book that if you can gently bring your worries and concerns out into the open and be prepared to listen to each other sympathetically, you are much less likely to build up major resentments that will ultimately cause you much more trouble. Don't sweep everything under the carpet 'until after the baby is born'. It will not be easier then. You will have broken nights and a demanding newborn and a lot less time to listen to each other. You may also have lost the opportunity for a happier and warmer pregnancy.

For those who do feel up to it, making love in pregnancy can be a liberating experience with freedom from contraception and worry about getting pregnant, or from the pressure to conceive.

A few people, however, find they lose interest in sex once it has 'done its job' and the foetus is growing inside. This seems, perhaps quite naturally, to be more common among women than men. Beware, however, of assuming this is true for your partner if she goes off sex in pregnancy.

My husband accused me of only being interested in sex to

make babies and not being interested in him. It was true that sex went up the scale of priorities when we were trying to conceive, but it was not true at all that I was not interested in 'non-productive' sex.

Sarah, sons 3 yrs and 3 m

If you have been trying to conceive for a long time, finally being pregnant may come as a relief. If sex had become a chore with pressure to perform at particular times, one or both of you may now want a break.

After about a year of not making much effort not to get pregnant and six months of positively trying to, I had decided I had a fertility problem. I started taking my temperature (to detect fertile days) and that put an enormous pressure because there was 'tonight's got to be the night'. You just had to do it. By the third or fourth cycle this was bad news. You just don't want to do it. It creates quite a lot of resentment and anger. It was getting quite heavy. I was really glad it only took eight months to get pregnant. Once I was pregnant there was a break. We both backed off. We were still physical – hugs and cuddles – but it didn't go further. Getting away helped. Every time we went away it was better. Sex had become a chore, another thing you had to do, and it took quite a long time to get back to it being an expression of your feelings.

Sammie, son 2 yrs

If getting pregnant has taken a long time, or involved complicated and uncomfortable fertility treatments, you may also feel very protective towards the longed-for foetus, and be afraid of doing anything that carries even the remotest possibility of harming it. Fear of hurting the baby is in fact quite common even amongst those with easily conceived, normal pregnancies. And men can be affected as much as women.

I was very concerned as a first-time mum about sex in the very early and late stages of pregnancy. I think you develop a very primitive protective mechanism and you want NOTHING to harm your cub.

Joanne, son 3 yrs, daughter 1 yr

We were both quite disturbed about what effect us making love would have on the baby. Eventually we bought some books and were reassured. He found it harder to get over the psychological barrier of 'there's a baby in there' than I did, which I found strange. I thought it would be me that was most protective.

Emma, daughter 4 m

We had quite a lot of confusion about the pregnancy and whether we could hurt the baby. In the end I bled and we weren't allowed to make love. I think it was a relief to both of us – we can't, we don't have to. The decision was taken for us.

Janet, sons 8 yrs and 4 yrs

We avoided intercourse in the first trimester because of a previous miscarriage...After that I did not worry about the baby, though it sometimes crossed my mind if ever sex was uncomfortable, but I would only have worried if I'd bled.

Jane, daughter 18 m

I was conscious of trying to be more gentle and less of the 'rough' passionate stuff.

Philip, daughter 7 m

We had needed fertility drugs to get pregnant. We had no sex during pregnancy. Not because we didn't want to, but because we thought it was safer for the baby – even though we had been told it was OK. We had no penetration, and not much else either. It wasn't hard to cope with because having a child was so important to us.

Roy, son 3 yrs

Such fears are, of course, particularly difficult where one of you is very worried and the other is not.

> Once we knew I was pregnant, my husband wouldn't come near me. He said it would hurt the baby. He'd read somewhere that orgasm could cause miscarriage and he wouldn't touch me at all. I was saying 'It's OK.' My sex drive really went up. It was so high, I've never felt so randy in all my life. I had to play with myself a lot. He played with himself too.
>
> **Sarita, daughter 1 yr**

You can of course seek professional reassurance for a worried partner, but if he or she remains really worried, it is probably better to find other ways of showing love until the end of the first trimester.

The nine months of pregnancy allow you to begin to adjust to being a parent before it actually happens. The process begins right from the time the pregnancy is confirmed. If you are able to see it in this light and help each other adjust, you will have a happier pregnancy and an easier time when the baby is finally born.

2

THE SECOND TRIMESTER

The Physical Effects

The middle section of pregnancy is when most women feel best. This may mean feeling especially well and 'blooming', or just feeling a little less ghastly. The most common symptoms of the first trimester should start to disappear or at least ease up a bit. Fatigue should become less overpowering and most women will stop being sick, though a few will not.

Breasts will usually become less tender, but extra sensitivity may remain. This can leave them still too sensitive for inclusion in love-making, or mean that gentle touching is extra pleasurable.

During pregnancy vaginal secretions usually increase and you may notice a mild-smelling whitish vaginal discharge. This is leukorrhoea and it is completely normal. Some men are put off oral sex by it, but it will not do anyone any harm.

Dark marks and stretch marks may start to appear on the skin. Some women get chloasma – dark patches on the face – and/or a brown line from the tummy button to the pubic hair. Both will disappear after the birth. Stretch marks may also start to appear on the tummy, legs or bottom. Gaining the right amount of weight may prevent some stretch marks, but even the most careful eater can get them in the end. Stretch marks will fade after the birth, though they do not disappear. Try to see them as honourable marks of motherhood!

By the middle of the second trimester you will almost certainly have a bump visible at least to you. You may be very obviously pregnant. For many couples the bump does not get seriously in the way of love-making until the third trimester but you may already need to change your love-making positions so as not to put weight directly on the pregnant tummy. With a smallish bump this can be done in the missionary position by the man taking all his weight on his arms, but side and rear entry positions are often easier. If you have not used these much before, have a look at Appendix B.

You may also find that you start to notice a hardening of the pregnant abdomen after orgasm. This is the uterus contracting but it is not a sign that you are going into labour and it is perfectly normal. If you have severe cramping pain after orgasm, however, it would probably be wise to consult your midwife or doctor before reaching orgasm again.

If you are going to have a time in pregnancy when love-making is particularly good, it is most likely to be now. In pregnancy, blood flow to the genital area increases and this can make it more sexually sensitive. Some women notice nothing, others find they reach orgasm more easily and/or that it is more intense. A few are turned on by almost anything.

> I recall vividly how incredibly sexy I felt when I was pregnant, a sensation that became more pronounced as the pregnancy progressed. I had never heard of this phenomenon before. In fact, I think I was under the impression that sexual relations ceased during pregnancy. It got to be quite a joke between my husband and I, as I could hardly cope with travelling on a train without becoming sexually aroused.
>
> **Margaret, daughter 10 yrs**

Sometimes the increased blood flow is less welcome. Pregnancy hormones can also make the blood flow back upwards through the body quite sluggish and this may make the whole genital area feel heavy and swollen. Some pregnant women get vulval or vaginal varicosities (just like varicose veins in the legs) as well as haemorrhoids (or piles, varicosities of the anus). Sexual arousal is likely to exacerbate any heaviness and may make orgasm more difficult and less satisfying, leaving you with a residual feeling of fullness.

You can help feelings of heaviness and discomfort due to varicosities by trying not to be upright all day. Lie on your side whenever you can so the blood does not have to flow uphill in order to leave the lower part of the body. Lying on your back will not help as the weight of the uterus can squash the main vein in the back.

Squatting, often recommended in antenatal exercise classes, is also not good for vulval and vaginal varicosities or haemorrhoids. If you are very uncomfortable a cold compress may help; for haemorrhoids there are various over-the-counter creams, both conventional and homoeopathic. Vulval and vaginal varicosities will disappear after the birth. Haemorrhoids may linger but should become much less troublesome so long as you avoid constipation.

Pelvic floor exercises (*see below*) may help relieve heaviness and reduce varicosities by encouraging blood flow back up the body. Some people believe the exercises can help protect the area from excessive damage during the birth and may help prevent postnatal problems such as the collapse downwards of the vagina and uterus (prolapse) and stress incontinence (leakage of urine when you cough, jump or – in a few cases – make love). A strong pelvic floor, and one that you can control, may also improve your sex life more directly. Tensing and relaxing the pelvic floor can add to the sensation of intercourse for both partners.

Pelvic Floor Exercises

The pelvic floor is the set of muscles that literally form the floor of the pelvis. The deep layer holds up the uterus, bowel and bladder. The outer layer forms a figure of eight around the vagina and urethra at the front and the anus at the back (*see Figure 1, page 20*). Not surprisingly, the pelvic floor comes under increasing pressure as pregnancy progresses and especially during labour and birth.

Try tightening the muscles around the genital area without tightening the stomach or buttock muscles at the same time. Do not hold your breath while you are doing it. If you find this difficult or cannot immediately feel your pelvic floor, lie on your back with your knees up (if you are already uncomfortable on your back, sit on a chair). Put your hand between your legs and try

Figure 1: The pelvic floor muscles

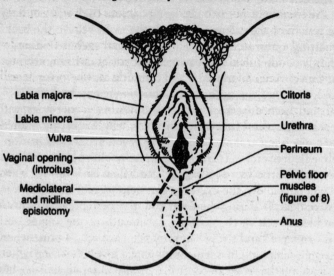

Labia majora
Labia minora
Vulva
Vaginal opening (introitus)
Mediolateral and midline episiotomy

Clitoris
Urethra
Perineum
Pelvic floor muscles (figure of 8)
Anus

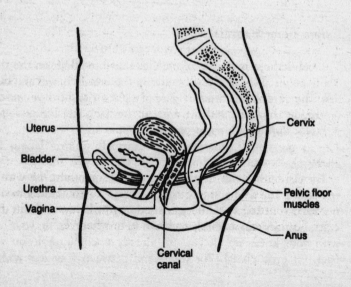

Uterus
Bladder
Urethra
Vagina

Cervix

Pelvic floor muscles

Anus

Cervical canal

again. You should be able to feel a slight pulling up of the pelvic floor. Alternatively, put two fingers just inside the vagina and try to squeeze them together.

It may take a while to be able to tighten the pelvic floor independently of other muscles or to feel that you are moving the area significantly. Keep trying. The more you do it, the easier it will get.

To strengthen the muscles, try the following exercises, repeating each one several times and doing the whole lot several times a day:

- Tighten the pelvic floor and lift as much as you can, then release repeatedly.
- Breathe deeply. Tighten and draw up the pelvic floor slowly on the in-breath and release on the out-breath.
- As above but hold the pelvic floor tight while you breathe out and in again before releasing on the next out-breath, or tighten and hold for a count of four and later for a count of 10 – but make sure you are not holding your breath.
- Imagine your pelvic floor area is a lift. Draw it slowly up and then lower it slowly down. Now imagine there are four floors this lift has to stop at. Draw up to the first floor and stop. Draw up a bit more to the second floor and stop and so on, and the same on the way down. You will probably find this difficult, but it is a very good exercise even if you cannot do it perfectly.
- Lift and release, then fully relax the pelvic floor at the end of letting it down. Try to imagine the baby's head coming down and breathe out as you try to release (though not push) the pelvic floor to allow the baby through.

Ideally you should be doing all the above, several times each, several times a day. Realistically, just try to do something. One way to remember is to link doing the exercises to something you do regularly – sitting at traffic lights, going to the lavatory (do them after, not before), washing your hands, or whatever.

Is Sex Safe?

By this time the pregnancy is established; the placenta is working and the main risk of miscarriage has passed. This is probably the safest as well as the most satisfactory time for sex. Do continue to listen to the woman's body, though. Don't do anything that is uncomfortable and if you have not been making love in the first trimester, take it gently at first.

You may have heard or read that cunnilingus (oral sex on the woman) is not safe in pregnancy. This is not true. This misconception arose from a handful of cases where the women died after having air blown into the vagina during pregnancy. If air is forced into the vagina under pressure it can go through the cervix, into the uterus and via the placenta into the bloodstream. If you do not blow into the vagina there is no reason not to have oral sex.

Complications That May Mean No Sex

INCOMPETENT CERVIX/CERVICAL CERCLAGE

If you have had cervical cerclage – a stitch to keep a weak or 'incompetent' cervix closed – you will probably be advised to avoid both penetrative sex and orgasm.

BLEEDING

A bleed in the second half of pregnancy – later second trimester and third trimester – is potentially more serious than earlier bleeding. About 50 per cent of the women who come forward with bleeding in the second half of pregnancy are eventually found to have either a detaching placenta (placental abruption) or a low-lying placenta (placenta praevia). For the other 50 per cent no clear reason is found. Both placental abruption and placenta praevia occasionally lead to serious haemorrhage (loss of a lot of blood), and placental abruption can cause the death of the foetus. So with late pregnancy bleeding it is vital to seek medical attention as soon as possible. You may be offered a scan to see what is happening with the foetus and to try to locate the placenta. Mild placental abruption will sometimes repair and bleeding stop, in which case you will probably be treated like someone for whom the bleeding is of unknown cause.

Sex certainly does not cause placenta praevia and the evidence so far is that it probably does not cause placental abruption either. There is, however, a possible risk in making love if you have either of these conditions.

A placenta that is over the cervical opening (over the os) or very close to it could theoretically be disturbed by both penetration and the contractions brought on by orgasm, particularly towards the end of pregnancy, and this could set off a bleed.

In the case of placental abruption, you may also want to avoid penetration and orgasm. Contractions of the uterus are thought to slightly and temporarily reduce the amount of blood (and therefore oxygen) getting to the baby. Normally this does not matter (the baby goes through far more during labour, and contractions during pregnancy are normal). But if the placenta is already compromised, it may be wise to avoid this.

PAIN
Abdominal cramping may be a sign of placental abruption, of late miscarriage (before 24 weeks) or, later, premature labour (24–37 weeks). It may be none of these, but it is probably sensible to try and find out what the pain is before continuing to have sex.

PREVIOUS LATE MISCARRIAGE
If you have had a late miscarriage in the past, you may want to discuss with your doctor or midwife why it happened and whether avoiding sex is a useful precaution in this pregnancy. If the previous miscarriage was due to something that is likely to recur, then the 'on the safe side' policy may be to avoid penetration and orgasm.

The Emotional Effects

You may now feel more confident about the pregnancy and more relaxed about making love. If you do feel like having sex and there is no medical reason why not, make the most of it. This may well

23

be the last time you both feel like it AND have time for it for quite a few months to come!

It is during this trimester that you will start to feel the baby move. For many couples, and perhaps especially for men, this is the turning point in really believing you are expecting a baby.

> My partner wasn't really 'involved' with the pregnancy until he could feel the baby move under his hand. He says he didn't think of it as real because it was hard for him to imagine the changes taking place almost daily in my body. I resented that, up until he felt the baby. Then he became excited and I felt I had someone to share it with.
>
> **Katie, son 2 yrs**

The bump may be becoming visible and you are perhaps now telling more people about the pregnancy. This should mean you get more help and consideration, and perhaps a seat on the train or bus (though don't bank on it!). For many there is also a feeling of pride as others express their pleasure and congratulations.

Such private and public recognition of the pregnancy is most often pleasing to both parents-to-be, but a few people find it difficult. You are, or your partner is, now identified as a mother-to-be. If you are happy with this role, it can be lovely. If not, the feeling of the baby moving and comments from others may be unwelcome.

If you feel very negative about the growing baby, you may need to address these feelings with your partner, friends, antenatal teacher or a trained counsellor. Strong and persistent negative feelings are almost always best dealt with now, before the baby actually arrives.

How you feel about the pregnancy rubs off on how you feel about yourselves and each other, and is very likely to affect your sex life.

> When I was pregnant, my partner became very awkward around sex, and if he could have got away with giving it up, he would have done (no chance!). He admitted to me that he thought/felt that his child was just the other side of my vagina and that he would damage it by having sex. Perhaps this also

had something to do with not finding a pregnant woman sexually attractive...He certainly had mixed feelings about parenthood.

Martha, daughter 3 yrs

In the second trimester, when I was feeling slightly better, love-making was a time of comfort and reassurance that Mike would be there to encourage, support and love me for my efforts (however they turned out) in labour. A time of oneness with each other and our new baby-in-the-making...I think my view of myself changed during my first pregnancy. I began to look at my breasts and think, 'these will feed the baby', to look at my abdomen and look forward to it growing larger and rounder. I was totally overcome by the magic of it all, the way that nature gets into gear and everything happens so perfectly. Such a complex process and yet so simply perfect.

Laura, daughter 8 yrs, sons 5 yrs and 18 m

Self-image is all-important to sex and a woman who is happy to be pregnant is much more likely to see her changing self as attractive and be comfortable about her pregnant sexuality. Some men find pregnancy a turn-off, because of the physical changes to their partners or because it represents the turning of lover into mother. Other men find it a turn-on, excited by the fact that together with their partner they are making a child and finding their partner's changing body particularly beautiful.

Women are very much affected by the attitude of their men. If the man finds his pregnant partner attractive and makes this known, she is much more likely to take a positive view herself. If he makes remarks about 'getting fat', she is likely to respond – or fail to respond – accordingly.

My husband found my pregnant body attractive, but because he has always teased me about being 'fat' I found this hard to accept.

Katie, son 2 yrs

Do bear in mind that women often put on some weight around the thighs, hips and face during pregnancy even if they are eating sensibly, and some women retain large amounts of water which make them look bloated and fat, even though they are not overeating.

Pregnant women get very mixed messages about their sexuality. While some magazines and books are telling them to make hay while the sun shines and they need no contraception, they are often being treated in antenatal clinics only as mothers-to-be rather than individuals. They may have doctors or midwives prodding their private parts as if they were public property, and you only have to look at most maternity clothes to get some very odd messages indeed.

> I have never understood why a normal adult woman is suddenly expected to want to wear little girl clothes with puffed sleeves and flowers just because she happens to be pregnant.
>
> Alexandra, daughter 3 yrs

Maternity bras, too, are often like Fort Knox, although the availability of more attractive maternity clothes has been improving and is likely to continue to do so.

Besides the issue of physical 'attractiveness', a few people are bothered by the now palpable presence of a third person. Men in particular occasionally say they feel uncomfortable or embarrassed making love in the 'presence' of the baby. They may describe it as 'feeling watched'. If you feel this, do try and talk about it. Like the problem of not wanting to make love to a mother, this is best dealt with now. You need to come to terms with sex as part of family life if your relationship is to flourish after the baby is born. It is especially important to deal with this one if the baby is ever going to sleep in your bedroom (more on this in Part III, Parenthood).

As pregnancy progresses, many women turn increasingly inwards. Even if they feel better in the middle months they may still not be very interested in sex.

> I felt well and was not yet too heavy, although a bit waterlogged, but I still didn't feel like it much. I was more interested in what was going on internally.
>
> Katie, son 2 yrs

26

Often, as the pregnant belly grows, the pregnant woman's world shrinks. She may become more home-based, less interested in the wide world, work and other people. Some men do not understand this or, if they do, feel a bit left out. This turning inwards is, however, a natural part of pregnancy and preparation for labour, birth and early motherhood.

Generally speaking, the more involved the man is in the pregnancy the more likely you both are to feel positive about it – and about your relationship and sex life. Whether or not you are having sex, remember that both of you may need extra reassurance that you are loved at a time of such change and so many future unknowns.

Women often want non-sexual attention to show them they are loved. Men on the other hand tend to attach love and sex more closely, often finding it difficult to separate rejection of sex and rejection of themselves.

When Carol was pregnant for the first time she totally lost interest in sex until well into the third trimester:

Our sex life became almost non-existent. I just was not interested at all. The very thought of it made me feel ill.

Carol regarded this as not unusual and of no great importance since pregnancy only lasts nine months. She loved her husband and did not see any reason why abstention from sex for a few months should be a problem. It was not until three years later that she discovered how desperately differently her husband saw it. This is Andrew's side of the story:

I still feel sickened and embarrassed that I could have reacted in such a one-dimensional and perhaps chauvinistic way to a set of circumstances that I guess, with the maturity of hindsight, were predictable. I knew that things would slow down a bit but sex dropped from two to three times a week to nothing. It was hell. I felt guilty for concocting situations or asking, and from a relationship that was as free and equal as any I had known before, Carol now held the ultimate power and it hurt badly. After the 'honeymoon' period of the first

27

trimester when everyone's feelings were up and down I expected us to pull together and be close, but no way...Carol made it very clear what she didn't want...there was no gentle let-down or explanation. Perhaps neither of us really understood what was happening, and this helplessness led to many hours of silent rage and frustration for me. I was getting shut out and I did not have the wild excitement of carrying a child to buoy me up during the down times...The only way I could get through 90 per cent of the normal passing of a day, that I could deal with the basic rejection of sex, love and romance (emphatically not just sex) was to lie to myself that I could handle the changes and that my next opportunity for togetherness may be more successful. After an eternity of rejections of any physical or indeed basic emotional togetherness the bad inside got so bad and I felt so alone that I was sure that our relationship was doomed, and it was in the back of my mind that it was only a matter of time before someone else showed me a crumb of attention or interest and I would not be able to reject it. I knew I wanted to stay in my marriage, despite all this, so I did not court or even plan an extra-marital relationship to substitute for what appeared to be irretrievably lost. Thankfully a fatal opportunity did not become available.

I was 24 and had always been demonstrative about my affections. I suppose at times I was oversensitive and insensitive. But I NEEDED reassurance from Carol...[and] I wanted to show her that pregnancy and motherhood had actually accentuated her looks and that to me she would always be my lover and girlfriend as well as a 'mother', and all its stereotypes.

This partnership not only survived but eventually flourished again, and their second pregnancy was completely different. Andrew again:

Carol was ill, sick, more tired, and wanted sex...By the second trimester I thought I had died and gone to heaven. It was spellbindingly different. We spoke more about why the first pregnancy had been so barren. Togetherness, closeness, friendship and yes, sex, had brought us together again which allowed us to talk frankly and cement our relationship. You can't talk intimately without togetherness – and we re-affirmed this.

The moral of this story, in case you haven't guessed, is to make sure you are clear that it is sex you are rejecting and not your partner, and not to rage silently, but speak up gently and talk things through. Even if you have always been brilliant at reading each other's mind, pregnancy is different and you may be misjudging each other terribly.

Practical Matters

It is probably at this stage that you will have to think seriously about how and where you are going to have the baby. This is the time to read the birth section (Part II) of this book and find yourselves a good antenatal class.

Do try to do as much of this as possible together. The more involved the man is, the more likely he is to feel positive about the whole thing, and the better your relationship (and sex life) are likely to be after the birth. Choose your antenatal classes carefully. There will be NHS classes at the hospital, but you may also want to consider National Childbirth Trust (NCT) classes, those based on the Active Birth Movement, or other independent alternatives.

If you are intending to breastfeed, make sure your antenatal class includes breastfeeding, or contact a breastfeeding counsellor for an antenatal session. Try to go to anything on feeding together. Even men who are very pro-breastfeeding sometimes have problems with jealousy and feeling left out after the birth. The more they know about it and can help their partners establish successful feeding, the less of a problem this is likely to be – and the easier time the new mother will have too.

Most antenatal classes allow time for discussion. This is a good place to bring up the subject of sex if you have questions or would like to know how others are coping. If you do not want to do this yourself, ask the teacher if it could be made a topic for discussion. If sex has already been discussed within the group during pregnancy, it will also be easier to return to the subject if you keep in contact with the group postnatally. Even if nothing of practical value is said, it often helps to know you are not alone.

The middle of pregnancy is also probably the best time to start to think seriously about what life will be like after the baby is born. There are all sorts of practical things that will change, and they will probably change much more than you expect. This may be especially true if you have always had a 50/50 split of everything. Pregnancy, birth and early parenthood affect men and women very differently and this can come as quite a shock to a relationship where you have previously led very similar lives.

Have a chat now about exactly what you each expect to happen. Areas you may want to look at include:

- Work outside the home: Who does it? When and how much? What limits on overtime? Who organizes childcare?
- Money: Who earns it? Whom does it belong to? What kind of bank accounts do you have? Will you each have some money you can call your own?
- The baby: Who is responsible for looking after it at night/during the day/in the evening?
- Household chores: if one of you is at home with the baby, is that person also expected to do everything else in the home? This latter is a classic case in which couples often have completely different expectations and do not realize it until it is too late and resentment is already riding high.

It is very common indeed for couples to talk about 50/50 splits in pregnancy that never happen after the birth. This is partly because you cannot know in advance what parenthood will really be like, but partly because couples are often rather unrealistic in their expectations. If one of you is at home with the baby during the day, for example, while the other is out, you will have to make a huge conscious effort if you want an equal split of childcare when you are both around, because the one who is at home most will almost inevitably become 'the expert'.

Talk to friends who already have children. Then talk to each other, trying to be as realistic as possible. At least get clear what you each expect to happen. This will at least leave less room for recrimination when you have to rethink the whole thing after the birth!

This may seem to have nothing to do with sex. In fact it has everything to do with sex. For example, a woman used to being in an office full of interesting adults who has just been alone with a whinging baby all day is unlikely to feel at her sexiest, especially if her man – who would never have expected her to cook supper when she was in her office job – arrives home asking where the meal is. (For more on this, see Part III).

3

THE THIRD TRIMESTER

The Physical Effects

As the pregnancy nears completion many women feel very heavy and tired. It is common to be sweating more than usual, find breathing restricted, need to pee very frequently and have a variety of aches and pains. It may be difficult to sleep and hard to get comfortable at the best of times, let alone to make love. Between two-thirds and three-quarters of couples give up sex in the last weeks of pregnancy, but some continue quite happily right up to the birth, sometimes despite common discomforts.

> Towards the end of the pregnancy I had carpel tunnel syndrome [numbness and pain in the hand], oedema [water retention] and quite a lot of pain. It was difficult to live everyday life, but sex was not too bad – at least you could lie down! My husband was very considerate and took his weight on his shoulders, etc. I remember having sex often in the late stages hoping to induce delivery.
>
> **Marion, daughter 3 yrs, son 1 yr**

Semen contains prostaglandins which are sometimes used in artificial induction. Some people think that intercourse may help start labour if you are already due.

Breasts sometimes get sore again at this stage in the pregnancy and a man who sucks his partner's nipples may get a taste of colostrum – sweet, thick yellow stuff that is the baby's first food. You may be advised to 'condition' or 'toughen up' your breasts for breastfeeding by expressing colostrum or rubbing the nipples regularly. If you do not like doing this, then don't. Research so far suggests it makes little or no difference.

Many women suffer from heartburn (acid indigestion) in the latter part of pregnancy. Since heartburn generally gets worse when you lie flat, you may want to consider more upright positions for love-making as well as sleep.

By this stage in the pregnancy, women often find lying on their backs makes them uncomfortable or light-headed. The weight of the baby can constrict the main vein in the woman's back and limit blood flow. If your blood flow is restricted then the baby's is too, so if you do feel odd, turn over. Lying on your left side should restore the blood flow almost immediately.

Is Sex Safe?

There have been various reports – several of them from the same research group – suggesting that sex in late pregnancy increases the risk of premature birth and other unwanted outcomes including detachment of the placenta (placental abruption) leading to severe bleeding (haemorrhage), amniotic fluid infection (chorioamnionitis), premature rupture of the membranes, and foetal distress. However, much of this research has been criticized for its methods, and the results are regarded as flawed.

Two scientific reviews of the research up to about 1990 conclude that there is no evidence that sex in pregnancy, including late pregnancy, is harmful and that to prohibit it in a normal pregnancy is 'wholly inappropriate'.

It may seem illogical to suggest that sex can induce labour when you are close to the due date, but not earlier. There is in fact no scientific evidence that intercourse does speed the start of labour. Even if it can, it is quite possible that it will do so only if all the other factors necessary for the start of labour already exist.

A large study in Jerusalem found that intercourse, including orgasm, right up to the end of pregnancy had no ill-effects, and a study by Wendy Savage and colleagues in London found no connection between late intercourse and foetal distress in labour. Research involving 126 women in Zimbabwe even concluded that the traditional prohibition of sex for those carrying twins is unnecessary.

Just as in previous trimesters, these results must be seen in context. They refer to pregnancies with no known complications and are observations of what couples did naturally. Only around a quarter to a third were still having sex in the last month of pregnancy. The idea that sex is safe in late pregnancy must carry the proviso that you do only what feels right and comfortable.

Complications That May Mean No Sex

Bleeding, placental abruption, placenta praevia, incompetent cervix/cervical cerclage, cramping pains: see Chapter 2.

PRETERM LABOUR (BEFORE 37 WEEKS)
If you have already gone into preterm labour in this pregnancy and it has been stopped with drugs, it is best to avoid sex altogether.

If you have had a preterm labour in a previous pregnancy but no problems this time then talk to your doctor or midwife about what caused the last one. If, for example, you were carrying twins and this is a singleton pregnancy, then the conditions that caused the last premature labour are unlikely to be repeated. If, on the other hand, you have an abnormally shaped uterus this will still be the case and you may be at risk of another premature birth. If the conditions that led to the last preterm labour are likely to recur, then the 'on the safe side' policy may be to avoid penetrative sex and orgasm in the third trimester.

PRELABOUR RUPTURE OF MEMBRANES
If your waters have broken, the baby is no longer fully protected from infection that may rise up the vagina, so it is best to avoid penetrative sex or introducing anything else into the vagina. Rupture of membranes may mean that labour is imminent, so if you are less than 37 weeks pregnant and do not want to go into premature labour, it may be safest to avoid orgasm as well.

The Emotional Effects

If the body is busy being pregnant, so is the mind. Some women simply do not feel like making love – nor do some men. The woman may be increasingly turned inwards, anticipating the birth, perhaps fearful of labour one minute and excited the next. She may be fed up with being pregnant and desperate to be able to lie normally again or to be holding a healthy child safely in her arms.

Men are obviously not physically affected by late pregnancy, but they are by now very aware of the baby who may be felt moving during love-making. A few find this inhibiting. The feeling of 'being watched' can get stronger, and fear of hurting the baby may return now that its head is perhaps 'just the other side of the cervix'. These fears may apply to both sexes, but if anything men seem more prone at this stage. So long as the waters are intact the baby is protected from both mechanical damage and infection and there is no need to worry.

Fears about labour and birth can also affect men. While the woman has obvious reasons to be concerned, men too may worry about how they will cope and what exactly they will be able to do to help. Do look at Chapter 4 on Fathers at the Birth.

One or both of you may find you are becoming very home-based. Curling up on the sofa with a cup of cocoa may seem like a much better idea than going out on the town or making wild, passionate love. The nesting instinct can be quite strong towards the end of pregnancy in both sexes. Heavily pregnant women are sometimes found halfway up ladders 'just trying to finish' or occasionally start whatever little project in the house suddenly seems vital to the well-being of the family. Or she may be out on her own because her man is frantically painting the walls before the baby is born.

Sometimes men get heavily involved in some non-baby-related project, often to the irritation of their women who can think of more useful, or more sociable, ways of spending the last weeks of pregnancy. Such engrossing projects are thought to be men 'creating' their own 'babies'. A few men go so far as to get ill in sympathy – or competition – with their partners.

Some weeks before our first child was due, my partner got ter-
rible backache. Then he got extreme fatigue and tummy
problems and he was very pale. He was laid up in bed for ages
and there was I hugely pregnant carrying trays of tea and toast
up to the bedroom. For a while the doctor thought he had
some post-viral syndrome. Then he came out in nettle rash
and we knew it was psychosomatic. In the second pregnancy
I joked that it would happen again and six weeks before due
date right on cue the backache came back. Each time, all the
symptoms disappeared within a week of the birth.

Michelle, sons 3 yrs and 1 yr

All in all, the last few weeks of pregnancy are for most couples not
a time when sex is at the top of their list of priorities. A few people who have worried very much about miscarriage and premature
labour, however, find sex more enjoyable after the 36th week. At
37 weeks a baby is officially 'at term' and even if sex were to start
off labour, the baby would not be premature.

If for whatever reason you are one of the majority of couples not
making love in the last weeks of pregnancy, try not to focus too
much on an expected quick return to 'normal' after the birth.
Equally, if your sex life has been especially good lately, do not
assume that this will continue soon after the birth.

As pregnancy progressed I grew less and less inhibited...The
night before I went into labour we enjoyed a marathon session. Nothing could have prepared me less for the complete
and utter change that followed.

Maria, son 10 yrs

The fact is that for most couples, and especially mothers, early parenthood is physically and psychologically exhausting and there are
a lot of things – including sleep – that take higher priority than
sex. So make the most of lie-ins, peaceful afternoons and early
nights (whether or not they involve love-making). It may be a
while before you have them again.

Summary of Part I: Sex in Pregnancy

- If you have no complications and you feel like having sex, there is no evidence that it is not safe to do so throughout pregnancy.
- Unless there is a medical restriction, follow your instincts. If it feels good for BOTH of you – do it. If it doesn't – don't.
- Talk and listen to each other. Don't assume you know what the other is thinking. This is a time of change and you might well get it wrong.
- If you have bleeding, abnormal discharge or excessive pain – investigate. If you are worried, you could abstain from sex until you have some idea of the cause.
- Many people worry about sex hurting the baby, or feel 'watched' by it in later pregnancy. The baby is well protected inside the amniotic sac and will not 'see' or mind what you are doing.
- Pregnancy may be a time of no sex or of more or better sex than ever. Both are normal. Most couples have sex less frequently, especially towards the end of pregnancy.
- If you are told not to have sex, make sure you know exactly what to avoid, why and how long the ban lasts.
- Ask straight questions of health professionals and insist on straight answers.
- Find a good antenatal class and go together. The better informed you are the less trouble you are likely to have, and the more involved the man the happier you are both likely to be.
- Talk as realistically as possible about what you expect your respective roles to be after the birth – and then be prepared to have a complete rethink after the baby arrives!

PART TWO

THE BIRTH

Giving birth to your first child, or being involved in that birth, is a rite of passage. It is an experience unlike any other. 'It is a lifetime's drama condensed into one day,' says Jane Hawksley, Relate counsellor and sex therapist, 'you will probably experience every emotion. You'll feel you've lived a lifetime.'

It is not surprising, then, that how the birth goes can have a profound effect on your sex life as well as on life in general. Birth is the culmination of your sexual relationship and is physically centred on the woman's sexual parts. It can be physically and psychologically elating, or occasionally it can be damaging.

The experience of childbirth can dramatically affect your attitude to each other and to sex itself. So it is well worth trying to maximize your chances of getting the kind of birth you want.

It is also vital to realize that once labour starts you cannot predict what will happen. You need to consider most eventualities and accept that in the event ideal plans may go straight out the window. The nature of birth is such that you cannot ultimately control it, but you can and should prepare for it. And the more of the preparation you do together, the happier the whole experience is likely to be.

4

FATHERS AT THE BIRTH

How you approach the birth as a couple will obviously affect how you feel about each other afterwards. Do you want to be together throughout or are you the sort of people who feel childbirth is a time for being with one's own sex?

There is no question about whether the mother is present at the birth – although there may be times when she wishes there were! But the father's presence is a matter of choice. Hopefully a choice you can make together.

In the last few decades the norm has shifted from one extreme to the other. Where the door used to be firmly closed on the father, now it is almost assumed he will be present – and some 90 per cent are.

Even during a Caesarean, the father is usually allowed to be in the operating theatre if his partner has an epidural anaesthetic and is awake. If she has a general anaesthetic the father will almost always be asked to wait outside.

For most couples the change in attitudes towards fathers is a change for the better. But do not allow peer pressure to force you into something that is wrong for you. If either of you has doubts about the father being at the birth, talk it over and decide what is best for you – and the hell with other people's opinions.

Fortunately, it seems to be relatively rare for partners to seriously disagree on this one. On the whole if the father wants to be present, his partner will probably want him there. If he desperately does not want to be there, she is quite likely to know that he won't be much help. One mother described how she told her husband to leave the room when she had to have a forceps delivery with her first child, and during her second birth she sent him to a football match.

If a man is really unhappy about being there, he may even be a liability. And in rare cases can have serious problems afterwards.

The blind assumption was that any right-thinking male would be at the birth. I was never really consulted. It wasn't my wife that drove me there – afterwards she said she didn't really feel very strongly about whether I was there or not. It was the assumption of others. I felt that as an ageing new man [aged 55] the least I could do was be there. It virtually killed my sex life and my wife and I subsequently separated.

I had chosen to regard that part of the female anatomy as a recreational area rather than a procreational one. I'm not that fond of bodily fluids anyway. It was a very messy, a very naked business. It doesn't allow for any of the sensibilities one might have. I ended up with two probationary nurses holding MY hands and soothing ME. The physicality of the birth – seeing the head emerge. It didn't render me impotent, but it rendered me virtually impotent towards my wife.

John, daughter 8 yrs

Experiences as bad as this are very unusual. For the vast majority of men, being present during labour and at the birth of their children is something they would not have missed for the world.

It was a fantastic experience. It didn't change the way I saw my wife at all. It was a long labour and at the end it slowed down so they got her to squat. I was by her side, holding her. Our son was born at 3 a.m. I got home at 7.30. I tried to sleep, but I couldn't. I went for a walk. I was walking on air.

Dave, son 2 yrs

An involved and supportive partner can also make a big difference to the mother.

My partner was fantastic. I could not have coped without him. He is not a man who normally lets his hair down particularly easily, but he let everything else go while I was in the worst part of labour. It certainly helped that we were at home with midwives we knew and not in a hospital full of strangers. He had his arms round my neck and encouraged me through every contraction for about seven hours. I didn't care who else was or was not in the room as long as he was there. When he finally said he had to go to the loo, I was desperate. I pleaded with him to get back before the next contraction. He had two minutes and he did it.

I felt very close to my partner after the birth. I felt he had really been part of it. I was the one in agony, but we really had done it together. He had sweat pouring down his face too…If I had been physically able, we would have made love within days. Needless to say, I wasn't and we didn't, but the feeling was there.

May, son 3 yrs

Christopher Clulow, director of the Tavistock Institute of Marital Studies, and himself a father, says sharing the birth of your children can be a strengthening experience for a relationship:

For many men this is a quite wonderful initiation into parenthood – something quite magical that can create a strong emotional bond. It underlines the joint project, being in there at the beginning, and it is extremely moving. Birth and death really put you in touch with your feelings; there is a heightened sensitivity. It is a lost opportunity if you can't share the really important moments.

Peter Walker, a teacher of postnatal exercises who also runs occasional fathers' groups, agrees:

What do you want to experience with your woman? Going out to clubs, wining and dining is all very nice, but labour and birth – these are REAL things. Childbirth is the major reality of life.

He adds however, that, 'You do have to WANT to be involved. If your heart is not in it, then it is no good. And the woman has got to want you there.' If either of you is still ambivalent, talk to other parents (of both sexes), bring it up at your antenatal class (preferably at a couples' session when fathers are there), and discuss it between you – repeatedly if necessary.

Women need to try not to rush or bully men into a decision, even though they may see this choice as a luxury they would like to have. The woman is going to do the hardest bit, and she may feel the least he can do is hold her hand and be there to know what she went through. Labour and birth are almost (some would say completely) unimaginable, so if you are NOT going to be present, do get a detailed debriefing from anyone who *was* present, as well as from your partner. This is really your only hope of understanding how she feels afterwards.

If you ARE going to be at the birth, it is important to get clear what your role will be. During labour your main job – and it is immeasurably important – is to support, encourage, and comfort your partner, and if necessary to be her mouthpiece, negotiator and advocate. You are not there to be part of the medical team, or stand permanently behind a camera (unless this is really what you BOTH want).

Men sometimes complain of feeling like a spare part at the birth. There may be times when you feel you are not doing anything, but you almost certainly are. Particularly in these days of high-tech hospital deliveries when you often do not know the midwife or the doctor, it is very important for a woman to know there is one trusted person there exclusively for her. A man who is not actually averse to being at the birth may find this reason enough to be present and never regret it.

I felt that anything I could do that would hasten the birth of a healthy babe by offering as much support as possible to my partner – be that physical ('rub my back there') or emotional ('just keep talking to me') – would justify my presence...In the event it was a long first labour. We arrived in the hospital with the expectation that my partner was two or three times as dilated as she actually was. The realization that despite the onset of real pain there was still hours to go was a harrowing moment to share with me – but surely a crippling moment to have had to face by oneself.

In early labour, when my partner was still having 'good' breaks between contractions when we could 'meet somewhere' and understand what each other was saying, I felt I was needed and valued support. And the more it went on and on the more she needed either my hand to squeeze or me reminding her to keep breathing, to keep looking at me, something, anything to remain sane. There was a particularly difficult moment when she pleaded with me to give her ANY drugs, she didn't really want the baby, 'you have it,' she said. When she was told it was too late for drugs, which she certainly understood theoretically, there was near despair in her stunned 'oh no' which I hope I managed to talk her through. In the second stage, frightened as I was by the visibility of the pain and angered by the bloody-mindedness of one particular midwife, I was too intent on willing/coaxing the crowned head into sight to do anything but stand there and be positive and encourage and ask for one more push, and, and...Eventually he did come out with his cord around his neck, and [when] we were convinced, seconds later that he WAS alive, we lay sobbing against each other, in happiness, love and relief.

Our love was not lost in labour. Perhaps it is easy to confuse love with feelings of physical/sexual intimacy. These were not helped by labour (and children), but our love and respect for each other grew in labour.

                                                        Luke, father of three

There is good research evidence to suggest that this sort of support during labour can actually improve the outcome for mother and baby, so if the father cannot be there, do try to find someone else who will support you/your partner through labour and birth.

When his first child was due, Peter Walker was very aware of his advocacy role:

It was very necessary that I was there. We had talked about things my partner wanted. The way women give birth is very, very personal – how, where, even when – and I wanted to be there to make sure she got what she wanted. I had to negotiate on her behalf.

In Peter's case this included persuading the midwives that his partner should not have to lie on a narrow hospital bed. His partner was having strong contractions and was not in a position to argue. He had to be very polite but insistent, and eventually the bed was moved and cushions provided.

It is not always easy to be diplomatic but do try, if only for your partner's sake. One mother said, 'My partner had a go at one of the midwives. He was right. But I felt, "No, no, don't do that – my life is in their hands." '

Even if you do not have to negotiate, you may need to ask questions on your partner's behalf and interpret some of what is going on. Make sure that the reasons for any examinations and procedures are given, and that results of any tests are offered to your partner as soon as possible. A woman in deep labour does not always hear everything (though never count on her not hearing!). Occasionally she may cut out all the unfamiliar voices of hospital staff and will hear only you or another chosen birth attendant.

Deep in labour, women may also say things that don't make sense, swear or be rude to people. This is especially likely during transition between the first and second stage, which is often the worst part of labour. If her wrath is directed at you, don't take it personally. She is probably in severe pain, frightened, exhausted, or all three.

Jane Hawksley says, 'When I was in labour, I told my partner to f– off at one point. Fortunately, it was my third baby and he understood. Men need to understand you are at the end of your tether.'

Experienced midwives will not be phased by any rudeness from a woman in labour. As one midwife put it, 'If she starts swearing – cheer – it probably means she is heading for second stage and it's nearly over.'

When she is not too deeply in labour, your partner may want to discuss with you any problems or decisions. If you know she felt strongly about something before labour, you may be able to help her through any problems that threaten to undermine her desires. But if she has really changed her mind, do not try to hold her to previous intentions. Nobody really knows what labour is like until they are in it.

If it is hospital staff who are pushing you into something you do not want, a written birth plan discussed with them prior to labour can be a useful negotiating tool (*see Chapter 5*). And the more you know about birth and hospital procedures, the easier your support and advocacy role will be. So it is worth reading the books and going to antenatal classes.

There is one other crucial piece of advice for fathers: Unless you desperately want to see the baby's head actually emerging, stay at your partner's head end. You will still need to be prepared for quite a lot of mess – which may include faeces and urine as well as blood – but you will be spared what a few men find to be a difficult image; that of their partner's genitals in unfamiliar form, or worse still, during a Caesarean, the inside of her abdomen. Such images seem to be at the root of many of the sexual problems occasionally suffered by men after the birth.

My husband thought the birth was the most revolting thing in the world. It was breech forceps with my legs in stirrups. It didn't bother me. I couldn't see anything. But it upset him a lot. He could see forceps going in and the baby's rear end coming out...The doctors were talking to him and making fun of him a bit, saying 'Come and have a look at this.' I think he felt a bit pressured. He really wanted to stay at the no-business end. He never said it affected sex, but I suspect it may have done.

Kay, daughter 2 yrs

Unless you have an emergency delivery with no midwife or doctor – in which case you will be far too busy to be shocked! – the 'business' end is not your problem. Your partner is most unlikely to be looking down there, and your most important job is to look after her.

Once the baby is born, you are, of course, there to share the first moments of your child's life. There may still be some crucial supporting to be done, especially if your partner has to be stitched, or if she or the baby need further medical attention. But when all the clearing up is over, the three of you should be left in peace for a bit of mutual admiration and recovery.

5

DECIDING WHERE AND HOW TO HAVE YOUR BABY

Where to Have Your Baby

Where you decide to have your baby can make a huge difference to how the birth goes. It is of great psychological importance that you feel comfortable with the place and the staff. How you feel can affect everything – even the apparently physical aspects of birth. Research findings show that women who are relaxed in their surroundings need less pain relief and recover more easily after childbirth.

You have a choice about where and how to have your baby. How much choice will vary from area to area. In most places, there will be at least two hospitals where you could give birth, each perhaps having a number of different schemes for delivery. These schemes vary in the amount of time spent at the hospital and in the balance of care given by the hospital doctors, midwives and your family doctor. Alternatively, you could book a home birth.

It is a myth that home birth is necessarily unsafe. Clearly, if you have a multiple pregnancy, high blood-pressure, a history of problems during labour or various other complications, it is advisable to have your baby in hospital. Otherwise a home birth, with experienced midwives and hospital back-up, is worth considering.

A thorough review of the scientific evidence on home birth recently concluded that there is no evidence to support the view that hospital is the safest place for all births. In the Netherlands, where almost a third of babies are born at home, the outcome statistics for mother and baby are some of the best in the world.

Precisely because hospitals and their staff are geared up to deal with difficult births, there may sometimes be a tendency to intervene too soon or unnecessarily, possibly turning what could have been a normal birth into a difficult one. Overall, the evidence suggests that home could even be safer for some low-risk births.

Besides the safety issues, where you choose to have your baby is all about feelings and instincts. Some couples find masses of technology and an operating theatre in the building reassuring.

> I knew I wanted a hospital birth. I wanted every bit of modern technology deployed on my behalf. It was partly because of a family history of stillbirth, but I have always liked hospitals and I knew I would feel comfortable there. I quite wanted to have only strangers with us in labour. It was something private between me and my partner and so the more faceless anybody else was the better.
>
> I had a very good birth. I insisted on being induced after my waters broke early. I knew I wanted an epidural and I had that early on. I asked for forceps to complete the birth.
>
> Kate, daughter 3 yrs, son 1 yr

Others find hospitals alienating and frightening.

> I went to look round a couple of hospitals and they just felt all wrong. Every one of my friends who had recently given birth (all first-timers) had had some kind of medical intervention. Hospital just felt like entirely the wrong place to have my baby. I knew I would have seen different people each time I went there and strangers again when I arrived in labour. Having no idea who would care for us in labour felt like playing Russian roulette with myself and my baby.
>
> We decided to have the baby at home with midwives we would know and would know us. We arranged good hospital back-up just in case. I had a long painful labour but nobody interfered; my partner was involved in a way I am sure he could not have been in a hospital; nobody told us what to do (unless we asked) except right at the end when it was necessary for delivery; and when it was all over we could all get into our own bed – the baby too – and go to sleep.
>
> Alice, daughter 2 yrs

Both the above were first births. Both women, and their partners, were sure of their decisions and both still felt they had done the right thing afterwards. You may not agree with either of them. Beyond the medical and safety issues, what matters is that you should be where YOU feel comfortable.

Since where you have your baby is likely to have a major effect on how you have it, do have a look at the next section and ask plenty of questions about the various alternatives before making a decision.

How to Have Your Baby

How you have your baby – flat on your back or standing up, with an epidural or drug-free, strapped up to a monitor or with periodic checks on the baby's heart – can all affect your subsequent physical and emotional health – and especially your sexual health.

Hospitals, doctors and midwives vary enormously in how up to date they are on the latest research and how much notice they take of it, so it is well worth getting yourselves as well informed as possible about what is likely to be best for you.

Minimizing Perineal Damage

Most physical sexual problems after birth arise from a tear or episiotomy (a cut along the perineum to increase the size of the vaginal opening). Nationally, episiotomy is done in about half of first births and over a third of all births. It was, until recently, a routine procedure in many hospitals, but most are now catching up with current research and are using episiotomy more selectively.

Routine episiotomy does not mean less perineal trauma and may even delay a return to sexual activity for some women. There are doctors who will still tell you that routine episiotomy protects against third-degree tears (into the anus) and that it prevents damage to the pelvic floor and so reduces the likelihood of postnatal problems such as stress incontinence (leaking urine) and prolapse (collapse of the vagina/uterus). You may be told it is better to have an episiotomy than risk a tear because a neat cut is easier to mend, and that routine episiotomy protects the baby's head from trauma. Research has found no evidence for any of these statements in full-term delivery.

Episiotomy should be used only to speed up delivery when this is really necessary – that is, when there is foetal or maternal distress (abnormal heartbeat or other signs of difficulties) or when the perineum does not seem to be stretching any more and is the only thing standing in the way of delivery. Episiotomy is almost always necessary for a forceps delivery – usually quite a large one – and it is sometimes used to protect the baby's skull in premature or breech births.

Adrian Grant, a leading healthcare researcher who has done a lot of work on childbirth says, 'A 20–25 per cent episiotomy rate would seem quite reasonable. Anything much greater would raise a question in my mind.' A recent study in Argentina also concluded that 'episiotomy rates above 30 per cent cannot be justified.'

You can maximize your chance of an intact perineum and minimize the risk of excessive damage by what you do and do not do during labour and the birth. Instrumental delivery generally causes more damage than spontaneous delivery, with forceps usually worse than ventouse. So anything that increases the likelihood of instruments being used also increases the chance of perineal trauma. Advice on what to do to help protect yourself is not always straightforward. You may have to strike your own balance between the advantages and disadvantages of any given action or intervention. And, of course, nothing carries any guarantees.

Try to avoid lying on your back. The shape of the pelvis means that if you do lie flat the baby then has to go slightly uphill to get out, and the pelvis cannot open fully as the sacrum (tail bone) is not free to move back. This may mean an episiotomy or tear is more likely. If you are lying flat on your back, the weight of the baby can also restrict the blood flow through the main vein in the back and reduce the oxygen supply to the baby. This increases the likelihood of foetal distress and intervention such as episiotomy, instrumental delivery or Caesarean section.

Unless there is a good medical reason why not, you should be able to move around as you wish throughout labour and delivery. If you need to lie down, which you will if you are very tired or have an epidural, try lying on your side.

Sometimes women are immobilized because of continuous foetal monitoring (monitoring the baby's heartbeat). Unless there is a complication, intermittent monitoring by the midwife or doctor with a stethoscope or hand-held ultrasound monitor is probably preferable. Research has found that intermittent monitoring done regularly by an experienced person is just as good in terms of the baby's safety, and probably better for the mother. It gives you freedom of movement, does not constantly distract staff, fathers and other birth partners, and is not open to such wide variations in interpretation. Research has shown that women monitored continuously are more likely to have medical intervention, including forceps and Caesarean deliveries, than those monitored intermittently, without any clear benefit.

Epidurals (anaesthetic inserted into the cavity around the spine to numb the lower half of the body) also stop you from moving around. A successful epidural is undoubtedly the most effective pain relief available, but it does increase the likelihood of instrumental delivery.

All pain-relieving drugs have their disadvantages. But so does going through hell. You have to balance things out in your own way, according to your own labour and situation. There is a now a 'mobile' epidural that allows you to walk around, but it is still very new and is only available in a few hospitals.

In the second stage of labour (when you are pushing the baby out) research suggests that you are likely to do least damage to the perineum if you are allowed to follow what your body tells you. Unless quick delivery is essential, you should not be told to push push push. When the baby's head crowns, however, advice from a midwife to relax or pant seems to help women give birth with minimum damage.

Some hospitals set a time-limit on the second stage of labour. The theory is that pushing for too long can cause distress to the baby. This sort of arbitrary time-limit can lead to unnecessary intervention to speed up the birth and therefore increased perineal damage. So long as occasional monitoring of mother and baby shows that all is well, and the baby is progressing towards birth, the second stage can be allowed to continue at its own speed.

Finally, if at any point during labour or delivery you are doubtful about what the midwives or doctors are doing, do ask. You are entitled to know what is going on and why, and if you are not happy about it, make your views (politely) known.

Stitching

Once the birth is over, any perineal damage may need to be stitched. The actual stitching should NOT be very painful. A survey by the National Childbirth Trust found many women suffered extreme pain during stitching. This should never happen. The injection(s) of local anaesthetic may hurt and it may all be uncomfortable. But if you have significant pain from the stitching itself, ask for it to be stopped immediately. Don't let anything more be done until you can be sure you have enough local anaesthetic and that it is working. Fathers and birth attendants may find this a moment for their advocacy role.

Stitching can also be a time when a bit of hand-holding and final encouragement is badly needed. Some women find it the last straw.

> I found being stitched up a bit of an abuse. Not because of the people doing it, just because I couldn't take any more. I had got through labour (without drugs) and pushed out a huge and lovely baby. As far as I was concerned I had done it now and I wanted my body to be left alone. Being stitched up was just one thing too many.
>
> Claire, son 2 yrs

Combined with how much of a cut or tear you have to start with, the way you are stitched is crucial to your early and happy return to sex (as well as life in general). The material and method used and the skill of the stitcher can all have a major effect.

The record of the medical profession on stitching women after childbirth is not, so far, very glorious. It used to be left to medical students on the grounds that the perineum was a 'forgiving area' that healed easily. Only very recently has more notice been taken of the real complexity of the task and the havoc that is wreaked with people's sex lives – and relationships – if the job is badly done.

Hospitals, and even individual consultants and midwives, vary in the materials and methods they use for stitching. With one exception (*see below*), absorbable stitches (those that should not have to be removed) have been found to be more comfortable in the days after birth than those that are not absorbed like silk and nylon.

According to current research, the best material for stitching is polyglycolic acid (trade names *Dexon* and *Vicryl*) which has been found to produce less pain than other stitching materials. It is more likely with this than with other absorbable materials that one or two stitches may have to be removed because it has failed to be absorbed and is irritating or 'tight'. But polyglycolic acid seems to be associated with fewer problems that require resewing.

There is some controversy about the stitching material glycerol-impregnated catgut, the most common version of which is called Softgut. One well-respected study associated it with more pain than other absorbable materials, both immediately after birth and during sexual intercourse months and even years later. The researchers recommended against its use. A recent piece of research did not confirm these results, but it was not nearly as good a study in scientific terms, so for the moment it would still seem sensible to avoid glycerol-impregnated catgut wherever possible.

There are two main methods of stitching. It can either be done with one loop and one knot per stitch (interrupted stitching) or as a continuous piece of sewing under the skin knotted only at each end. The latter, known as continuous subcuticular stitching, has been shown to be the more comfortable, both immediately after the birth and three months later. It is however the more difficult method, so whether the outcome is really going to be better for you will depend on whether there is somebody able to do it properly.

Skill is of course the other major factor in successful stitching. Although experienced perineal stitchers are not always the best (old habits die hard and are not always good ones), some experience certainly helps. Medical students are no longer supposed to stitch the perineum after birth – although it does occasionally happen. But junior doctors (known confusingly as Senior House Officers or SHOs), sometimes with almost as little experience, still do a lot of stitching.

If you think the person stitching you has no idea what they are doing, you can ask for the consultant, registrar or senior midwife. Alison, herself a medical student, still has problems due to incompetent stitching after her son was born four years ago.

> I was stitched by a junior doctor who quite clearly didn't know what she was doing. She kept saying, 'I'm not sure if I'm doing this right,' and asking my husband where the bits fitted! It still isn't right now. I have since seen an SHO make a total mess of stitching a woman because he had never done it before. In the end the consultant had to be called, all the stitches were taken out and the whole thing had to be done again.

This is, of course, another time when fathers or other birth partners need to be prepared to represent the new mother. She is very unlikely to be able to do it all herself.

It is increasingly common for midwives to do the stitching. This will, hopefully, be a good thing. It should mean that the new mother is stitched as soon as she is ready (i.e. once she has had a chance to draw breath, cuddle the baby and perhaps give it a first feed) rather than having to wait for a doctor to be called from elsewhere in the hospital.

Midwives are more likely to have been with the woman through labour and birth and therefore to see her as an individual. And most midwives are women, possibly (though not necessarily) giving them a head start in caring for another woman's sexual and 'marital' future.

It may be that there will be much less stitching in years to come – either because skin will be left unstitched or because other ways will be found of holding the wound together.

One very small study concluded that hisoacryl – a glue-like substance – was more comfortable than stitches two days after the birth. But much larger and longer-term studies are needed before this material can be generally recommended.

Some midwives and doctors have already stopped stitching smaller tears, and are treating deeper wounds by stitching the muscle layer but leaving the skin layer to heal itself. A group in Ipswich is doing a large trial to evaluate this method; results are expected in late 1995.

Birth Plans

Making a written birth plan can do a lot to help you get the kind of birth you want. Good midwives and doctors will take notice of what you say, and may pay extra attention on the day to your particular areas of concern. Research has shown, for example, that women who express strong feelings about not being cut or tearing may have a greater chance of avoiding it.

Writing a birth plan also focuses your own attention on the practicalities of labour and birth. And it brings out any differences in your own and your partner's views and assumptions before it comes to the crunch.

Discuss the plan with your midwives, doctor or consultant and try and get them to agree to it. This may bring out information about hospital routines that you would not otherwise have known and reduces the room for disagreement when you are in labour.

Birth plans, like rules, however, are made to be broken. Very few births happen as written. Once labour starts, you may find you feel very differently about the whole thing. Changing your mind – especially about such subjects as pain relief – is very common, especially with first births. Try not to worry about it.

If you do feel strongly about something, inform yourself well and then do not be afraid to be quite forceful. But do try and keep your birth plan and any necessary negotiations friendly and polite. You need the support of staff, especially if you are asking for something that is not the normal routine.

Before writing your birth plan you may find it helpful to read the sections on birth in a couple of the pregnancy and birth 'handbooks' (recommendations in Further Information at the end of this book) as well as Chapter 4 and the earlier sections of this chapter. The list below may help you think of what you want to include in your birth plan.

- What kind of birth are you hoping for? ('natural'/intervention-free/maximum pain relief/hospital/ home, etc.)
- Do you have any arrangements or preferences about midwives and doctors?
- How do you feel about episiotomy and tearing?
- What are your views/hopes about pain relief, including epidural?
- Do you have any strong views on:
  induction
  positions during labour and birth
  presence or absence of the father/other birth attendants
  use of water in labour/birth
  food and drink during labour
  type of monitoring
  internal examinations (frequency/position)
  forceps and ventouse
  who should be given the baby and how soon after birth
  third stage of labour (syntometrine)
  length of labour and artificial acceleration?
- If you have to have a Caesarean, do you have views on type of anaesthesia, presence of father/birth partner, etc.?
- Do you want the baby always with you after the birth or should it be sent to the nursery if you are very tired?
- Are you intending to breastfeed? Do you want to feed soon after birth? How do you feel about formula supplements? Do you want to demand feed?
- Is there anything about you (medically or otherwise) or your partner that your carers ought to know?

Contraception

You might be surprised to find this under the birth section of this book. But, believe it or not, you are quite likely to be asked about future contraception within a few days, or even hours, of the birth! You may find this deeply irritating (and you would not be alone) since sex is not likely to be the main thing on your mind. But the professionals are determined to get to you before you go home. The next time they will see you routinely is at six weeks, and by this time some couples have already had sex at least once (and once is enough to conceive again).

It can certainly be argued that the system needs changing so that health visitors or visiting midwives discuss contraception at a more appropriate time – some do, but this is usually on top of the earlier discussions.

> Contraception was not an issue for us – but it seemed to be for everyone else. I felt like a congenitally irresponsible idiot as I was told about contraception by 1) midwives 2) obstetricians 3) home midwives 4) doctor 5) health visitor. And none of them spoke to or asked to speak to my husband!
>
> Katie, son 2 yrs

Being prepared can make these enquiries less irritating. If you know exactly what you want to do about contraception, you can get rid of someone quite quickly. If not, you will be able to use them more effectively to get the information you want. If you make a decision before the birth, though, do be prepared to change your mind afterwards when you may feel quite differently.

If you have questions, write them down, and if the nurse or midwife gives you any instructions about your contraceptives make sure you get those in writing too. Your mind is likely to be on other things in the first days and weeks after the birth.

If you have questions about sex after birth, other than those specifically about contraception, a family planning nurse is often a good person to ask. You may find the person talking to you is an ordinary ward nurse or midwife, but you can ask (gently!) if they have special FP training. Such training does involve some general aspects of sexuality as well as contraception.

If you are fully breastfeeding, this will offer some contraceptive protection. If you are feeding the baby at least four-hourly day and night with no supplements (even water), your periods have not returned and your baby is under six months old, then you are 98 per cent safe (as good as most methods of contraception). Very little research has been done into how much protection a lower level of breastfeeding offers, so unfortunately you cannot rely on it.

Although your periods may not have returned, you can never be sure you are not fertile because you will ovulate BEFORE your first period arrives. Hence the concern about choosing contraception soon after birth if you do not want another pregnancy too quickly.

Medically, the ideal contraceptive in the first postnatal weeks is probably the condom, but it is not acceptable to everyone and your choice has to be a balance between medical and personal considerations.

The following run-down on contraceptives is not intended to be comprehensive (see *Further Information*). This section is specific to the problems of returning to contraception after childbirth.

Please note also that the percentages given are for use over a year. So 98 per cent safe means that two couples out of a hundred using the method for a year are likely to get pregnant.

Condom (Male)

In many ways this is the ideal contraceptive for the postnatal period – at least from the point of view of health. It is readily available over various counters (or free on the NHS), carries no health risks and even protects against infection. The only possible side-effect is allergy to the spermicide or lubricant, which can be solved by trying different condoms or buying a non-allergenic brand with no spermicide and non-allergenic lubricant.

The condom can have no effect on the baby and can be used as soon as you feel up to making love after the birth. Used properly it is 98 per cent effective, although studies of general usage have produced pregnancy figures of between the correct-use 2 per cent and 15 per cent.

If a man finds it difficult to have or keep a strong erection, then the condom may not be suitable, since sperm can leak out if the penis is not fully erect. A man with erection difficulties may also find the business of putting it on too much of an interruption.

Some men, with perfectly strong erections, object to condoms because of loss of spontaneity. Fatherhood will bring greater obstacles to spontaneous love-making than this. If the woman feels strongly against other forms of contraceptive – most of which are less effective, less tried, or carry some risk of side-effects for her or the baby – then perhaps he could read up on contraception a bit before putting the case against condoms too strongly. His partner could also try offering to put the condom on as part of foreplay.

In the postnatal period when the woman may be slower to become aroused and slower to reach orgasm, the slight slowing effect the condom may have on the man can also be quite useful!

The Female Condom

This is a relatively new contraceptive, which is a loose tube designed to line the vagina. It has a ring at the closed end which is pushed up to the top of the vagina to help hold it in place, and a ring at the lower end where it opens out around the vulva. The female condom has all the same health advantages as the male condom but is less tried and tested.

The Family Planning Association says that, used properly, the female condom should be as effective as the male condom, but there is little research so far. One trial in the US found a failure rate of 13 per cent in six months (i.e. potentially 26 per cent over a year), but the FPA suggests this is partly due to people not yet having learned to use it properly. 'User-failures' include the penis going up beside the condom instead of inside it.

Cap and Diaphragm

If you have used a cap or diaphragm before the birth, it is important not to assume that it will be as effective afterwards. You may need a new size after giving birth, and will have to wait at least six weeks before you have a fitting. This is the time it takes for the vagina to regain its muscle tone.

The need for a fitting can be a disincentive to a woman who is still trying to reclaim her body after childbirth. One mother said that, even nine months after the birth, she still could not bring herself to face the internal examination required to get a new cap. In the meantime, she and her partner used condoms.

Like all barrier methods, the cap and diaphragm do not affect breastfeeding. But do take care not to leave them in for too long. The cap or diaphragm needs to stay in for six hours after intercourse to be effective, but should never be left in for more than 24 hours, as there is a small risk of toxic shock syndrome. This is when bacteria enter the bloodstream through tiny cracks in the vaginal wall; it is more likely when something (cap, diaphragm, Tampax) is left in the vagina.

Used properly and with spermicide (as they should always be), caps and diaphragms should be 97–98 per cent effective. Studies in the general population have found failure rates between 2 and 15 per cent.

If the woman is not very interested in sex after the birth, the cap and diaphragm may not be the ideal contraceptives. They require her to think ahead and act on the prospect of sex, which may be the last thing she feels like doing. This may not improve either the likelihood of sex or its chances of success when it happens.

'The Pill'

What we usually refer to as 'the pill' is the combined (oestrogen and progestogen) pill. This is not suitable while you are breast-feeding because it can reduce your milk supply. It is also not rec-ommended if you think you have, or think you may have, postnatal depression. Otherwise, you can start taking the pill 21 days after the birth. You will need to see your doctor or family planning clinic, and all the usual health checks and side-effect warnings apply. Also, if you are planning to have another child soon, you may like to consider research findings that some women take a little longer to become pregnant after coming off the pill than when stopping other forms of contraception.

If you are returning to the pill, whether immediately after the birth or after some months (or years) of breastfeeding, you may find your old pill does not suit you as it once did. Pregnancy and childbirth can change your hormonal make-up, and you need to be aware that you could react differently even to a pill you have taken before.

Progestogen-only Pill (POP)

Breastfeeding women can take the progestogen-only pill (POP) and it can be started from day 21 after the birth, although a later start at perhaps five weeks may mean less irregular bleeding. The POP does not affect the milk supply and, although some of the hormone is bound to go through to the baby, this is not believed to do any harm.

The POP has to be taken within three hours of the same time every day, so is only suitable if you can keep yourself to this strict routine – which may be hard in the unpredictable postnatal period. It is less effective than the combined pill, but if you are breastfeeding the contraceptive effect of feeding and the POP together give almost 100 per cent protection. Once you have stopped breastfeeding you can return to the combined pill if you want to.

The FPA warns that the POP may be less effective in women weighing over 11 stone/154 lb. Even if you are not normally this weight, you may have some extra left after pregnancy and birth, so do check. If you are fully breastfeeding this will probably make up for any possible reduction in effectiveness, but talk this through with your family planning adviser.

There are fewer restrictions on who can safely use the POP than there are on the combined pill, but it does have its own restrictions, risks and possible side-effects. One side-effect is very common; periods are likely to become irregular and you may get spotting between main bleeds. A few women stop having periods at all. Other less common side-effects include weight gain, headaches and loss of sexual urges. If you do start the POP soon after birth, bear in mind that symptoms may be due to either proximity to birth or to the POP. Unlike the combined pill, the POP has no effect on your likelihood of getting pregnant quickly when you stop taking it.

Some doctors rarely prescribe the POP and may forget that it exists as an option. So if your doctor says you cannot go on 'the pill', because you are breastfeeding or for any other reason, ask specifically if you could use the progestogen-only pill.

Injection

The most common injectable contraceptive is Depo-Provera, lasting 12 weeks. There is also Noristerat, lasting eight weeks. These are injections of progestogen, and possible side-effects include heavy menstrual bleeding, weight gain and mood swings – and of course you are stuck with any problems for the duration of the injection's effectiveness.

Injection is best given six or more weeks after the birth. It may slightly increase production of breast milk, but not to the extent of causing problems. Fertility may, however, take up to a year to return after the last injection wears off.

Implant

The only implant currently available in the UK is Norplant. It is another progestogen method of contraception, but this time delivered by six small rods implanted in the woman's arm. It can be implanted six weeks after the birth, although there may be waiting lists for implantation. It lasts five years.

As Norplant is new, any long-term effects relating to breastfeeding are not known. The FPA says there is no reason to believe it will be different from other progestogen methods, which are considered safe. Eighty per cent of women get irregular bleeding in the first six months with Norplant, and there may be other side-effects.

The implant can be removed at any time and its effect is stopped immediately. Fertility returns within 48 hours, but

Norplant would not normally be given to anyone wanting contraception for less than three years.

The Vaginal Ring

This is not available at the time of writing, but should be in the next year or so. It is another progestogen method of contraception, this time delivered via a ring placed high in the vagina, which can usually be put in six or more weeks after giving birth. It is in many ways similar to the POP, but because it is in the vagina the dose can be lower, and it can remain in place for up to three months. It can be removed at any time, either permanently or for up to three hours if, for example, one or both of you prefers it not to be there during love-making. If the ring comes out it can be washed and put back. The arrival of the ring on the market has been delayed by the discovery that some women develop a red area of skin inside the vagina where the ring sits. This now has to be fully investigated before the ring is made generally available.

IUD (Intrauterine Device, Coil)

If you want to use an IUD and you are breastfeeding, make sure your family planning adviser knows you are breastfeeding. Breastfeeding women have a slightly higher risk of the IUD perforating the uterus during insertion. Breastfeeding causes the uterus to contract and a smaller uterus is more easily damaged. Try not to breastfeed for three hours before the IUD is to be fitted and be sure that the device is put in by someone with a lot of experience.

You normally need to wait six weeks after the birth before having an IUD fitted, and it is probably best not to do it if you are still sore, since inserting an IUD can be uncomfortable even normally. Very occasionally an IUD will be fitted earlier, but only if the woman is not breastfeeding and the person putting it in is very experienced.

The earlier an IUD is inserted after giving birth, the greater the chance that it will be expelled from the womb – that is, pushed out by natural contractions. If this happens, you need to use alternative contraception until you can go back to your doctor and get another one fitted.

If you have had a Caesarean, it may be advisable to wait three months before having an IUD put in. This is to ensure that the wound on the uterus is fully healed, otherwise there is a small risk of the IUD being incorporated into the scar tissue of the wound.

When in place, the IUD is between 97 and 99 per cent effective. If you get pregnant with the IUD in place it increases your risk of miscarriage, so if you want to keep the baby you need to get the IUD removed as soon as possible. If you do not miscarry, however, there is no evidence that the baby will be damaged in any way.

Sterilization

Sterilization, whether male or female, is permanent contraception that cannot generally be reversed. Although it may be tempting to 'kill two birds with one stone' and have a sterilization while in hospital for the birth, this is not a good time to make decisions as drastic as this. You can have no idea how you will feel about another baby once the current one is established or if (God forbid) something were to happen to him.

Female sterilization done at this time is also more likely to fail. The blood supply to the Fallopian tubes is greater just after birth, so there is a chance the tubes (which are cut or sealed in the sterilization) may mend themselves.

If you are planning a sterilization for urgent medical reasons (for example if another pregnancy would endanger the woman's life), perhaps the man could have the operation (a vasectomy) instead since he will have been physically unaffected by the birth. A vasectomy is also safer, requiring only local anaesthetic, and more effective, with a failure rate of only 0.1 per cent.

Natural Methods

The most effective natural system involves using all the various indicators of the stage in a woman's cycle, including temperature and cervical mucus as well as anything else you notice. The method requires commitment to daily checks and the ability not to have sex when you could get pregnant (or to use another contraceptive at these times). Recent research suggests that, done properly, natural contraception can be as effective as the pill.

It is not a method you can learn adequately from a book or leaflet. You need to see a trained natural family planning teacher and work out how to use the system best for your own personal cycle.

Ovulation kits now available for predicting fertility in those trying to get pregnant are not suitable for use in contraception. Apart from being very expensive, they only predict ovulation 24 hours before it happens. Since sperm can survive inside the womb for up to three or even five days, the sperm could already be sitting there waiting for the egg, before you even know you are about to ovulate.

If you have used natural methods of contraception in the past, there is no reason not to continue to do so after a baby is born, although you will be dealing with a less predictable situation until your menstrual cycle returns. And since pregnancy can change your hormonal make-up, the signs you were used to before you were pregnant may not be exactly the same afterwards.

If you have not used natural methods before, this is not the best time to learn. You have no established cycle, no 'normal' against which to measure what is happening. If you like the idea of the method, however, you could contact one of the organizations that specialize in it with a view to learning more once your cycle returns to normal.

The type of contraception you use can be quite important. If you are anxious about returning to sex, or your sex drive is low in the early weeks and months, a contraceptive you are relaxed with can make a big difference. Confidence in your chosen system is also important since if you have a traumatic birth, fear of another pregnancy can interfere with a return to a happy sex life. This may be true for men as well as women, and it is worth discussing this if either of you feels uncomfortable with your choice of contraceptive or thinks anxiety is interfering with your desire for sex.

If there is any disagreement about the kind of contraception you use, it is perhaps a good rule of thumb that whoever wants sex most should give way to the one who is finding it harder to get interested or aroused. This may be something very obvious like the choice between a cap (which she has to remember) and the condom (which has to be put on him) or more subtle; for instance, if you have always used the pill, but after the birth the woman feels very strongly against hormones going through to the baby, it might be sensible for a man who wants an early return to relaxed sex to agree to use a condom for a while.

Once you are at home, contraception is handled either by a Family Planning Clinic or by a GP surgery that offers family planning. It may be worth checking whether your doctor has training in family planning, since the fact that a family planning service is offered does NOT guarantee that the doctors or nurses have any special knowledge. To be considered trained in family planning a doctor should have an FPA Certificate, a Joint Committee on Contraception Certificate or a Diploma of the Faculty of Family Planning from the Royal College of Obstetricians and Gynaecologists. Nurses should also hold some qualification.

If you find your doctor unhelpful or unsympathetic you can go to an FP clinic or you can register for family planning with another GP. There are quite tight restrictions on which GP you can register with for general medical care, but you may be entitled to register elsewhere for family planning. So if a friend has a more sympathetic or better trained GP, see if you can sign on there for family planning, staying with your own doctor for everything else.

6

THE EARLY DAYS

This is a time of recovery and the beginning of adjustment to a new life – the baby's and your own. If this is your first child, remember those irritating people who kept looking at your pregnant tummy and saying, 'Ooh, life will never be the same again'? They were right. It may not be better or worse, but it will be different.

Sex is certainly not on the menu immediately after birth, and what follows may appear to have little to do with sex directly. But it does. The inclination to make love is, not surprisingly, closely linked to how you and your sexual parts feel or have recently felt. The way you care for yourself, your baby and your relationship (and the way they are cared for by others) in the early days can make a lot of difference to how easy it is to return to a sexual relationship later.

As the father, try to take as long a time off work as you possibly can. It is worth establishing your place in the new family. You need to get to know the baby and to understand a bit about his care. You will be badly needed by your partner and you may yourself need time to adjust to being a father.

Tiredness

You will be exhausted – especially the mother. Probably more exhausted than ever before. Get as much rest as you can in the early days when hopefully the baby will sleep quite a lot, if unpredictably, and when you may have more help than you will later. In the first few days try not to allow too many visitors to add to your exhaustion. Limit numbers and the time they spend. Fathers are often the best people to mediate and if necessary gently lay down the law to visitors.

If you feel terribly weak and fatigued it is possible that you are short of iron. Anaemia (lack of iron) is not uncommon in the postnatal period, so try and eat plenty of iron-rich foods (e.g. egg yolk, liver, kidney, shellfish, red meat, spinach, spring greens, legumes – such as peas, lentils, chick peas and kidney beans – cocoa and carob, soya products, and dried fruit). If you still think you are anaemic, ask your community midwife or GP for a blood test to check your haemoglobin levels.

(A lot more on tiredness in Chapter 8!)

Caesarean

After a Caesar you will spend 5–10 days in hospital. Post-operative pain can be severe and you should be provided with adequate pain relief. The doses given and the types of drugs used are considered safe for the baby, so do not struggle on without. Your baby needs you to be comfortable enough to get to know him.

Once you get home you need to remember that you have had a major abdominal operation as well as coping with the emotional business of giving birth. You may have escaped some of the trauma to the vaginal and perineal area, but if you have had a long labour before the Caesarean you may have sore genitals as well, and be extra exhausted. You need to take it very easy indeed, and get as much help as possible. Even lifting the baby may be difficult at first, and heavy lifting should be avoided completely.

Much of what follows will apply to you just as it does to any other parents, but you may also want to talk to other couples who have had Caesareans and read a bit about it (*see Chapter 8 and Further Information*).

Care of the Perineum

Unless you had a Caesarean section with little or no time in labour, your genital area is likely to be sore. If you had an episiotomy or a sizeable tear, you will have stitches which are almost certain to cause some discomfort. Even with an apparently similar wound, the level of pain women experience varies enormously from mild discomfort, that requires nothing more than understanding, to extreme pain.

If you are having trouble sitting comfortably, there is a special shaped cushion called the Valley Cushion that can be bought (though it is expensive) or hired through the NCT. As its name suggests, it has a dip in the middle to take the pressure off the perineum. Hospitals used to use, and recommend, rubber rings (like children's swimming rings) but these were found to interfere with the blood flow from the area. The Valley Cushion is thought not to do this.

Oddly enough, both warmth and coolness may give short-term relief from perineal pain. Use either or neither – whatever makes you feel most comfortable. You can cool with crushed ice wrapped in a clean pad, witch hazel (also on a clean or sterile pad) or tap water, though ice should not be used too much as excessive cooling can slow down healing.

Warmth can come from a warm cloth or a bath or shower (not too hot). Various things have been recommended to put in baths. Salt and Savlon have both been found to do neither harm nor good. If you don't want anything in your bath, don't bother. If you do, use whatever you find helpful or comforting.

Some women gain relief from homoeopathic Hypericum and Calendula tincture (10 drops in 200 ml boiled and cooled water applied to the sore area) which is thought to promote healing. Arnica 30 (in tablet form; some Arnica creams should not be used on open cuts) may ease bruising, and Bellis Perennis 30 is recommended for a severely wounded perineum.

If you are in a lot of pain you can buy Lignocaine local anaesthetic in a water-based gel or spray. Get a plain one without steroids or anything added. Steroids in this context may do more harm than good. The gel is applied locally to wherever it hurts. It is short term and will not affect a breastfed baby. Epifoam, though still sometimes recommended, is best avoided, as it may delay healing.

If putting local anaesthetic on the wound is not enough, paracetamol – up to 3g a day – can be taken by mouth. If you are breastfeeding, anything you eat can go through to the baby, but paracetamol is not thought to do any harm. Jennifer Sleep, a very experienced midwife and researcher in this field, says simply, 'It is not great for the baby if you are so screwed up with pain that you can't breastfeed properly – everything is a balance.'

Do use paracetamol rather than aspirin for pain relief, as aspirin has more potential side-effects for mother and baby. And beware of pain-killers containing codeine as they can cause constipation, which is well worth avoiding with a perineal wound.

Many women find the prospect of their first post-labour bowel movement very worrying. Some get so worried they keep putting it off. This will lead to constipation and then they really do have a problem. Try to eat sensibly after the birth – plenty of fruit, vegetables and liquids – and opening your bowels should not be painful. Don't worry if the first bowel movement takes a few days to happen. This is normal. Just don't hold back.

If it makes you feel safer, use your hand with a (clean) pad of lavatory paper or similar to hold the wound while you do it. If you do get constipated, try a natural laxative like prune juice. Failing that, a mild laxative from the chemist is probably better than hard pushing. If you are breastfeeding, stimulant laxatives such as senna (Senakot) and castor oil are best avoided because they may give the baby colic and/or diarrhoea. Bulking laxatives are probably best, and several are considered suitable for breastfeeding women: Regulan, Isogel, Fybogel, Celevac and Normacol. Osmotic laxatives such as Lactulose (often prescribed for constipated babies), and magnesium hydroxide (Milk of Magnesia) and magnesium sulphate (Epsom Salts) are also safe, but they may take a couple of days to work. If yours is an immediate need for help in emptying your bowels, you are probably best off with a simple glycerin suppository which can be bought over the counter.

Keep the wound clean and dry. Change sanitary towels regularly, and in hospital make sure baths and bidets are cleaned thoroughly before you use them. This can be easier said than done if the staff are unwilling and you do not have a visitor to enlist. If you are stuck, a shower is probably safer than a bath or bidet. Alternatively you could just wash your wound and wait until the bathroom is cleaned (or you are at home) to wash the rest of you.

To wash your wound without bathing or showering, pour or splash a bowl or jug of warm water front to back (so no faecal material gets washed on to the wound).

Try not to rub the wound. Dab it dry with a clean pad of tissue and ignore advice to use a hair-dryer. This can over-dry the wound and may be a source of infection.

If at any time you think your wound may be infected – if it is very red, raw, swollen, smelly or pus-like – contact your midwife or doctor as soon as possible.

Average, uninfected episiotomies ought not to give you serious trouble beyond the first week or two, but they quite often do. If you are still having trouble by the time of the six-week check, or if it hurts when the doctor starts to examine you – do say so. He or she needs to know how sore it is.

Some women worry that they are irreparably damaged or horribly mutilated 'down there'. They rarely are. It is true that in most cases the perineal area will not look, or perhaps even feel, exactly the same after childbirth as it did before. But it should not feel uncomfortable or fail to function in any way. If you are concerned about the shape of things, have a look with a mirror and, when it is no longer painful, have a feel around.

To speed up the 'normalization' of the perineum after birth, you can also do pelvic floor exercises. Though it may sound ridiculous, it is worth having a gentle try at these exercises as soon after the birth as possible. Some physiotherapists say within hours. Try very gently lifting the pelvic floor (*if you have not done this before, see page* 19). If it hurts, stop. It is more likely that you will feel no effect. This does not necessarily mean your muscles are doing nothing. It may just be that you are still a bit numb after the birth and cannot feel it. So long as it doesn't hurt, you can keep lifting a few times in a row, a few times a day until you can feel what you are doing (*then, see page 109*).

One of the theories behind recommending early pelvic floor

exercises is that other damaged muscles have been found to heal more effectively if they are being used. In a used muscle, the fibres in the scar tissue seem to develop in line with those in the surrounding tissue, whereas in an unused muscle they develop all higgledy-piggledy. A muscle with all its fibres in line works better, with potential benefits – in the case of the perineum – in comfort, successful urine retention and sex.

Haemorrhoids (Piles)

Sometimes the discomfort after birth is not only (or not at all) due to the perineum, but to protruding haemorrhoids. These can usually be felt as soft little lumps, sometimes described as a mini-bunch of grapes, sticking out of the anus. Use a bit of *KY Jelly*, or similar, and gently push them back inside. Take care not to get constipated.

If they are very painful you could ask to see an obstetric physiotherapist within a few days of the birth (*see Further Information*). There are various creams – both homoeopathic and conventional – that may be helpful, and you can use the same local anaesthetic gel recommended for the perineum on your anus if necessary.

Haemorrhoids may go within a few weeks. Even if they do not, they should at least become manageable.

Breastfeeding

The first time you put your baby to the breast – which should be as soon after the birth as you feel ready – you may be shocked by just how hard she sucks. It shouldn't actually hurt, it is just very strong. Don't worry, this won't damage your breasts and it shows your baby knows how to get her food.

Establishing feeding is one of the main efforts of the first few days and it is not always plain sailing. It can be especially difficult if you have had a Caesarean and the baby has to be positioned to avoid the scar, or if you get unhelpful or conflicting professional advice.

The father has a vital role. His support, or lack of it, can make or break his partner's confidence and therefore her ability to breastfeed. He can also be of practical help by reminding her what was said in antenatal breastfeeding classes when she is struggling to get a feed going. Be tactful: 'Didn't they say...?' is always better than, 'You're doing it all wrong.' But your help can be invaluable.

It is vital to learn, with your baby, how to get her latched on properly. This is the best – and only proven – way to avoid sore nipples and other feeding problems.

The simplest way to do this is to lie your baby horizontally on her side so she is looking straight at the breast. Then make sure her mouth opens wide and goes right round the areola and not just over the nipple itself. The nipple alone cannot take the strain and will eventually get sore. The baby may also get frustrated. The milk ducts are under the areola and the baby needs to put pressure here if she is to feed successfully.

If you find this difficult or if your nipples start to get sore, talk to an experienced breastfeeding counsellor as soon as possible (*see Further Information for contacts*). While you are sorting out the baby's position, you may want to help your sore nipples as well.

Nipple shields are not a good idea, at least for any length of time, because they can suppress the milk supply. There are various creams and sprays on the market. A few have been scientifically evaluated (including Masse cream) and found to be of no benefit.

Some women swear by *Camillasan* or calendula ointment. It is possible that these may help by treating sore and cracked nipples much as lipsalve treats sore and cracked lips, but they have never been scientifically tested. Do not use soap on your nipples, and dab rather than rub them dry. Do not use a hair-dryer on them as this can over-dry the skin.

When the milk comes in (to replace the colostrum) around day four, you may also find your breasts engorged (over-full). This can be very uncomfortable and you may want to express (by hand or with a pump) just enough to relieve the pressure. Try not to express too much or too often as this only stimulates milk production.

Emotional and Baby Blues

Birth is in one way a very ordinary experience – most women go through it, and these days most men play a part in it. But it is also quite extraordinary – a real rite of passage and something that can be very traumatic. Most women, and some men, have a few days of feeling quite shocked, especially after a first or unexpectedly difficult birth.

Some homoeopaths recommend taking a single dose of Staphysagria 10 M on the fifth day after the birth, or before if the 'baby blues' set in, to help with the emotional impact. A second dose can be taken two weeks later if the blues or depression have not lifted.

The 'baby blues' usually arrive on day three to five and can make the new mother very low and weepy. It happens to most new mothers and shouldn't last more than a matter of days. Nobody knows what causes the blues but it is perhaps a combination of hormonal changes, release of tension, exhaustion and other emotional factors.

Women can become very easily upset, and may find themselves crying without really knowing why. They may be over-sensitive to things that are said by relatives or medical staff, and are more worried by minor problems than usual. 'Blues' mothers may feel very tired and lethargic most of the time, and find it quite impossible to stop crying or cheer up. Sometimes the crying is not all misery:

> I only had to look at my son and I cried. It wasn't sadness. More a mixture of disbelief, fear, joy, love, vulnerability. I was just emotionally overwhelmed by his very existence and everything that went with it.
>
> **Chrissie, son 2 yrs**

New mothers with the blues need understanding, a good cuddle, to be allowed to cry and NOT be told to pull themselves together. They need plenty of rest and a chance to talk when they want to. New fathers may also need to talk.

One or both of you may need to go over the birth (perhaps several times); to talk about what happened and why. It is a way of sorting it out in your mind and getting over it.

You may also need to mourn a lost you – the freedom, perhaps the career, the individual you have left behind. Do mourn if you need to. It is an important part of being able to move forward. It is a bit like moving house. You may be sad to leave the old place, but allowing yourself a tearful goodbye does not mean you do not want to move or that you will be unhappy in the new house.

It is vital not to suppress feelings at this stage. You may think it is inappropriate to be miserable when you have this lovely baby (and some insensitive soul may even say so). It is not inappropriate and it is very important that you allow yourself and your partner time and space for guilt-free expression of your feelings – whatever they are. If you bottle up the negatives now you can be storing up depression for later.

Keeping in touch with people you met in antenatal classes can give you an extra circle of understanding friends to talk to. It is often harder for men to get a chance to talk outside the home. If your antenatal group gets together as couples or has a fathers' group, do try to go. Men are also often less forthcoming than women. But if you can pluck up the courage to open a topic, others will almost certainly follow. Sharing the problems of early parenthood really does halve them.

Time

It may seem at first that you will never again have time to do anything but baby care again – let alone make love.

My partner came home one night and we launched into the complex nightly bathtime routine we had been taught by the midwives. About halfway through my partner said 'I don't see how we are ever going to have a decent supper again, never mind do anything else.' It did feel like that. It took us about another week to realize babies do not need to be bathed anything like every night and that this complex routine was almost all unnecessary. Supper returned and eventually so did a few other things.

Natasha, son 3 yrs

Parents do have less time to themselves, but the early chaos and confusion does not last. The frills will go and you will get everything else down to a fine art. Life does not return to anything like it was pre-parenthood, but life does return.

Summary of Part II

- The birth of your first child is a rite of passage that can affect your relationship, sex, health and day-to-day life.
- Do your homework – as much as you can together – and decide what suits you: home/hospital, technological/natural as possible.
- You can and should prepare for labour and birth; you cannot, however, completely control it.
- Doctors and midwives vary enormously in how much notice they take of research. It is down to you to know what you want.
- Write a birth plan and do not be afraid to make your views known, before and during labour and birth.
- Use contraception as soon as you start making love again after the birth unless you are prepared to risk becoming pregnant again.
- The early weeks after the birth are likely to be emotional, exhausting and chaotic. A few days of baby blues are normal. Don't expect a quick return to your pre-pregnancy sex life, but remember the postnatal period is temporary.

PART THREE

PARENTHOOD

7

IS THERE SEX AFTER BIRTH?

Is there sex after birth? 'Isn't the answer just "No"?' said one mother with a 12-month-old daughter. She had good reasons for feeling like this. She had had a difficult birth and her episiotomy scar still hurt when she tried to make love; she and her partner had found it hard to adjust to being parents; she was working part-time from home with negligible childcare; and she was permanently exhausted. Parenthood just did not seem to her to be compatible with what she once considered a normal sex life. Now, two years later, she and her partner have two children. There *is* sex after birth – eventually.

Some couples sail through it all, of course. There are those who give birth, wait a few weeks and resume a flourishing sex life without a hitch or a grumble. If this is you – enjoy it. You are lucky – and there are not that many of you.

There could perhaps be more people who recognized themselves in this description if we had more realistic expectations. Whether your sexual relationship is, or feels like, a problem in the postnatal period has a lot to do with what you expect.

One couple will say, 'We didn't have any problems. It was only seven or eight weeks before we resumed intercourse. It was a little sore to start with but we took it gently and very soon everything was fine. We don't do it as often as we used to, but then we have rather a lot else to do these days.'

While another might say, 'It was ghastly. It was almost two months before we could make love and then it hurt. We still don't have sex as often as we did.'

If you expect a baby to be born one day and have passionate sex the next (or even the next week, or month), then you are heading for trouble. If you think about what pregnancy and birth are really like, what they do to a woman's body and the incredible results they have, it is hardly surprising that the period after a baby is born is one of intense physical and psychological adjustment, when everything needs to be taken gently.

Many women (and a few men) go off sex partially or completely for months after a baby is born. This may not be ideal, especially in today's sex-expectant society, but it is normal. And it is temporary.

Sometimes – especially if the birth experience has been good and you have both been very involved – you may find sexual interest is strong in the first days or weeks (when, unless you are very lucky, you can't do much about it), but tails off by six weeks, just as it starts to be a physical possibility. This can be very frustrating, so don't allow your expectations to rise too high, too early.

Some women say they are just too exhausted for sex, too engrossed in the baby, simply physically and emotionally used up. Others describe it as like a switch being flicked that just turns off all sexual interest. It makes sense if you think of it biologically. Nature (if one can talk of such a thing) is interested in you caring for the baby you have got, not in you making another one.

You can try to ease exhaustion and give yourselves more time together, but if libido is really gone you may just have to put your sex life on hold for a while and keep reminding yourselves that this won't last for ever.

Be sure to nurture your relationship in other ways. The key is to keep it intimate and affectionate, with plenty of non-sexual physical contact. Then when interest returns, the sexual relationship can just slot back into place. This is much easier said than done, of course, and we will come back to it in Chapter 9.

When your sex life does return, it may not be exactly as it was before. The idea that you will 'get back to normal' can be misleading. Some couples do go back to something very like their pre-pregnancy sexuality, but for others things are different. Sometimes they are better. Quite a lot of parents who have passed the period of postnatal adjustment say the quantity of sex is down, but the quality is up!

How Long...?

The usual advice nowadays is to resume sex 'whenever you are ready'. A few doctors still advise waiting until after the six-week postnatal check. This is out of date. If you feel like having sex, or doing something sexual, before six weeks, go ahead – but do be sure that you BOTH GENUINELY feel like it. If either one of you does not want to, don't push. Early pressure, be it from your partner, professionals or friends (and they all happen), can be very counterproductive.

If imposing a six-week rule on yourselves helps, then do it. But do not fall into the trap of thinking that six weeks is some magic time at which suddenly everything will be fine and ready for action. 'When you are ready' means exactly that, and for many people six weeks is not nearly long enough.

It is usually the woman who takes longer to recover – for obvious reasons – although men also sometimes need a while to get over the business of birth. Research studies show anything between about 30 and 60 per cent of couples have 'resumed' sexual intercourse within six weeks, and the great majority have done so by three months. This means they have done it at least once. It does not mean they are necessarily doing it regularly or that they always find it satisfactory. This may take a bit longer. Some couples do not have sex at all for six months or more, and over half of couples are not making love as often as before they were pregnant, even a year after the birth.

There is a very wide range of 'normal' in terms of sexual adjustment after a baby and you should not allow yourselves to be pressured – in either direction – by other people's, or your own, assumptions.

We started off with non-penetrative sex and that was fine, except that I began to think one OUGHT to be able to do penetrative sex. We tried just before the six-week check so that we would be able to answer when the doctor asked if it was OK. There are lots of reasons to have sex, but to please a doctor really isn't one of them.

IS THERE SEX AFTER CHILDBIRTH?

We didn't do it again for ages. Now we have patches of better and worse. Sex is far from regular. If I had more time to worry about it I'd be worrying about it. I would also be worrying about it if I thought it was seriously affecting our relationship.

You don't have to have a sex life, but I have these sneaking suspicions that one OUGHT to have a sex life. Then I think, this is ridiculous, I'm trying to be Superwoman.

Victoria, daughter 9 m

Victoria and her partner, incidentally, got their sex life back on track a few months after the above was said. They are now expecting their second child.

It does not in itself matter how often you do or do not have sex – or if you do at all – so long as it is not upsetting either of you or damaging your relationship. Magazines, books, advertisements and even friends may say, or imply, that somehow you SHOULD be having sex. There are no 'shoulds' about it. Except that you should both be reasonably happy.

If lack of sex or a change in your sex lives is affecting your happiness or your relationship, then clearly it matters a lot and you need to look at what can be done about it. This may be to find a way of making more space for your adult relationship and having more sex, it may be a matter of adjusting the way you make love, or you may need to establish alternative ways of showing love and affection and accept the reality of little or no sex for a while.

Whatever your situation the most crucial thing is communication. Even minor problems can spiral out of all proportion if there is no effective communication. If you are not used to talking intimately or talking about sex, this can be difficult, but it is absolutely vital.

I was so determined to reassure my husband of my continued love and desire for him that I didn't feel I could say no to intercourse. But with the baby waking two to six times a night, I felt as though my husband and son were conspiring against me to stop me sleeping.

Going to bed exhausted at the end of the day, I would gratefully accept my husband's offer of a cuddle, as I needed reassurance of his love and support, of course. But this turned into full sex-most times. I didn't feel I could turn him down as I feared he would feel rejected and on the few occasions I did refuse I felt so guilty that I'd toss and turn until I suggested intercourse!

I was pregnant with my second child by the time my first started sleeping and after the second birth I was again exhausted and reluctant to have sex, but having it all the same, and doing my best to have orgasm to keep the man happy while feeling sheer rage inside.

The crunch came when I told my husband that I felt as if he was attacking me when he put his hand on my breast. The whole tale came out and he has been wonderful and understanding and patient ever since. I don't know why I didn't talk to him before.

Vivien, mother of two

If you can keep talking and keep cuddling (without it carrying the assumption of a continuation to sex) small problems will sort themselves out and bigger ones will be easier to overcome. Most problems in the postnatal year are temporary, but they can cause longer-term problems if they are not dealt with together in a sympathetic way.

The First Time

Making love again for the first time after a baby is born may come completely naturally and be no problem at all. It may equally raise some anxieties in advance and some unexpected reactions at the time.

Choose a time when you are not TOO tired and agree what you will do if the baby wakes or cries. Don't be surprised if love-making is a little messy (leakage of milk if you are breastfeeding, or blood if you do it very soon after the birth). It may – even should – also be done with less abandon than usual. Her breasts may be sore and if she has had a tear, cut or bruising of the perineum, you will want to be particularly careful on entry.

After a Caesarean birth, you may want to make love in a position that keeps his weight off the scar. She can go on top or you could try her lying on her back with her legs over the edge of the bed so that he can kneel on the floor between her legs, putting no weight on her at all (*see Appendix B*). Be warned also that in the first three months or so after a Caesarean, orgasm may be painful because it is contracting the wall of the uterus which is still healing.

Keep your expectations realistic and take it very gently. This is, after all, only the first time.

Fear of being hurt, or of hurting her, is often one of the barriers to making love again. It is a very reasonable fear, though it often proves unfounded.

> I really wanted to feel close and sexual with my partner, despite a lot of discomfort with my stitches. We took a lot of time and care as I was fearful of the pain. But it was great.
>
> **Lena, son 9 m**

> I remember being very scared of making love after my first baby was born. I was scared of penetration. I was like a girl making love for the first time, only more scared. I was very scared of pain and of being a different shape and size. I was worried he would say it was not the same any more and that I would feel it was not the same any more. When we actually did it, there was no pain, and size was not a problem. It was all OK. I had no fears after the second birth.
>
> **Sharona, daughter 3 yrs, son 9 m**

Size and shape are common worries. It is true that if you try making love soon after the birth, you may feel that it is a bit cavernous inside. Don't worry. This is not the permanent shape of things to come. This feeling usually goes in a matter of weeks as the muscle tone returns, and you may be able to help this along with pelvic floor exercises (*see Chapter 8*).

Pain is a different matter. Make sure your partner understands your fears. Talk about it before you try making love, and agree that if it hurts or is uncomfortable, you will say so immediately and stop.

This needs to be seen as a trial run, so if it doesn't work nobody feels cross or rejected. You can always try again in a few days.

> I was a bit worried about the scar and a bit dry. But I wasn't afraid it would hurt. I could always say stop if it did.
>
> **Dawn, son 1 yr**

> When we first tried to make love at three weeks, I had no pain externally, but internally it felt almost like another contraction. I almost regretted doing it. We waited another week then it was OK.
>
> **Lea, daughter 1 yr**

It can be useful to have a tube of *KY Jelly* to hand since dryness is often a problem with first intercourse (*see Chapter 8, Dryness*). Make sure you use it to help rather than replace natural arousal. Even if you don't think KY is absolutely necessary, it may give you confidence by reducing initial friction on entry.

There is nothing wrong with a bit of alcohol either if you think it will help, but don't overdo it. Men in particular need to stay in control if they are to be very gentle and to be able to stop if requested.

Some couples find it helpful to do something non-penetrative before trying intercourse itself, and women may want to masturbate, or at least explore a little by themselves, just to regain confidence.

> I think at about three weeks we first had some kind of sex. I was nowhere near ready for full sex, but we gave each other an orgasm (manually). I can't remember if we used KY or just spit. I think spit. I remember saying afterwards, 'Well, the system still works.' We didn't try full sex until six weeks and I'm sure it was that bit easier because part of the system had already been tested.
>
> **Jennifer, son 2 yrs**

If your first attempt at intercourse is painful, uncomfortable, or just not very satisfactory, don't panic! Satisfaction is most likely to be a matter of time, relaxation and confidence. And some discomfort during sex soon after giving birth is, unfortunately, not uncommon. It usually disappears by itself or there may be a very simple reason for it – like dryness – that can be quickly sorted out (*see Chapter 8*).

Occasionally intercourse causes a return to bright red bleeding after you had settled into a minimal dark discharge or stopped bleeding altogether. As long as there are not vast quantities, this is nothing to worry about. Just wait a few days before you try again. If there is a great deal of blood, you should of course consult a doctor.

Besides the possible physical concerns, you may find that one or both of you feels strange about sex after birth. Some couples feel 'naughty', like teenagers snatching time, or even virginal.

> I felt very virginal, possibly from such close contact with a pure newborn being and I didn't really want to sully that.
>
> **Joyce, four children 13–2 yrs**

There may be odd feelings about having sex as parents (do parents have sex?). One woman said it was as she imagined making love to one's brother might be. Quite commonly, first love-making may bring back aspects of the birth. These may be pleasant, unpleasant or just there.

> My first orgasm after the birth (which was not accompanied by penetration) brought the image, even feeling (though none of the pain) of the baby's head coming out, not of anything going in. I thought of Sheila Kitzinger and her description of birth as orgasmic (which it certainly wasn't at the time). It was very odd, though not at all unpleasant. I think it only happened the once.
>
> **Chrissie, son 2 yrs**

> We first tried to have intercourse after the six-week check. It was fairly awful. During sex all I could think about was the birth. The pain and the fear of damaging my perineum

again...The first time was definitely the worst...After that, the violent mental images of the birth gradually faded.

Lucia, children 3 yrs and 1 yr

After each birth, the first few times we made love I would burst into floods of tears. It brought it all back. It wasn't nasty exactly. I just found being entered again, opening up there again, traumatic. After four or five times I was fine.

Jenny, sons 3 yrs and 1 yr

After our daughter was born, when we were in the early stages of making love I would have an image of Catherine splayed out in the delivery suite. During the actual labour there may be several hours with the woman splayed out like that and various doctors coming in to look. I found the image slightly troubling, a bit of a problem at first. But it wasn't enough to put me off completely and it faded with time.

Nicholas, daughter 1 yr

All these reactions to sex – before, during and after first making love – are perfectly normal and they almost always disappear quite quickly. Very occasionally they may linger; this is dealt with in Chapters 8 and 9.

8

PHYSICAL HURDLES

Tiredness

Tiredness can ruin your sex life, and babies are unbelievably tiring. Physically and emotionally they are more exhausting than almost anything else; certainly anything that would be regarded as normal. Even by a year after the birth 20 per cent of women say tiredness is interfering with their sex lives.

The demands of a new baby are tough enough if you start off fit and well rested, but you don't. You start with late pregnancy, labour and birth. The term 'labour' is well chosen. Giving birth is very hard work, and can leave you shattered.

Just as you are trying to recover, you are thrown into a whirlwind of constant demands 24 hours a day, a learning curve as steep as any you are likely to encounter, and a period of physical and emotional adjustment that goes to the heart of your personality and relationships. As if this weren't enough, the mother may have a painful perineum (and pain is itself exhausting) and be struggling with a rocky start to breastfeeding. The whole thing is far more exhausting than most non-parents could ever imagine.

I have climbed mountains overnight, worked 36-hour shifts, had only a few hours' sleep night after night on some project or other, but I have never, never been as exhausted or desperate for sleep as I was in the first few months after my son was born. I can remember sitting with him in the middle of the night on the verge of tears – or in tears – begging him silently to sleep so that I could sleep as well.

Claire, son 2 yrs

> Even when we have the desire [for sex] we usually can't do anything about it. Either we're doing something with the baby, or, once she is asleep, we're exhausted. We just collapse into bed. These days she is in bed by 9.30/10.00 and sleeps through the night, but I'm still exhausted. I don't have the emotional energy for sex. Terry's routine hasn't changed as much as mine, and he used to be up until 1.30 in the morning. But even he is exhausted. At least it is both of us. There isn't one wide awake and amorous.
>
> Emma, daughter 4 m

In general, the woman is likely to be more tired than the man. Even if looking after the baby is really shared equally – which is extremely unusual – she starts well below the zero line, with birth to recover from. If the baby is breastfeeding, that can in itself be tiring and means that she will be doing most of the night duties. Many 'new men' intend to get up and stay up with their partners while they breastfeed, but this rarely lasts more than a week. After all, what is the point of sitting there watching? Especially when you have to be *compos mentis* at work in the morning?

It certainly does not make much sense for there to be two walking zombies in the house, but beware the job argument. It may hold water for a while, if the woman is at home, has plenty of help, an easy baby and a guaranteed chance to sleep during the day. Otherwise, unless you have a very exceptional job (an airline pilot perhaps) this argument is highly suspect. There is hardly an office or manual job in the world that is more demanding than looking after young children all day (let alone all night as well). Most people who have tried both employment and full-time parenting – or perhaps who juggle a mixture of the two – are quite clear about which is easier.

> I go to work to relax. It is much much easier to be at the office than at home. And that was true even when I only had one child. Work is much more focused, you only have one job. At home you constantly have to think of what to do next, and it is lots of jobs. You aren't just expected to look after the child or children. You end up doing everything from taking in the

dry cleaning to dealing with the gas man at the same time.

Office colleagues do not generally throw tantrums or put bowls of baked beans on their heads. Adult society is much more predictable. You can make time to think. It is much less tiring because it is so much calmer and more ordered.

Marsha, daughter 4 yrs, twins 2 yrs

An overtired parent is no better at her or his job than a tired employee is at hers or his. A reasonably well-rested parent is vital to the emotional and physical well-being of your children, so, if you value your children, protect the carer's sleep at least as much as the breadwinner's.

If you are bottle-feeding, there is no reason why night duty should not be shared from the beginning, and even breastfed babies may need something other than milk in the night. Changing, walking, rocking or otherwise settling can all be done by the non-feeding parent.

If, for whatever reason, your partner is doing most or all the night parenting, you need to be constantly aware of how tired she (or occasionally he) is going to be. You may be tired too, but the one with constantly broken nights will be more tired, regardless of what you do during the day. Rest is not just a matter of number of hours in bed. Having to force yourself awake at regular intervals can leave you feeling quite desperate.

Exhaustion is very destructive. It leads to slowness, misjudgement, bad temper, excess worry and a host of other negatives – not to mention loss of interest in sex. Clearly it is not helpful for both of you to feel like this. But the less-tired partner needs to be very understanding of those symptoms of exhaustion that are less than pleasant to live with.

Having differing levels of tiredness can also lead to conflict of interest. What a well-rested, or even moderately tired, person wants from life may be quite different from what an utterly exhausted person wants – particularly when it comes to going to bed.

> When my children were young, I regarded sex quite simply as a waste of good sleeping time.
>
> Caren, four children 22–16

> When our son was a baby I would go to bed thinking, 'If I'm lucky, I can just get two and a half hours before he wakes up hungry.' Then my partner would start cuddling up and I'd think, 'Oh no, I can't bear it. If I accept this my sleep is probably down to an hour and a half.'
>
> Sally, son 3 yrs

If you have a sleeper for a baby, the problem of exhaustion may start to improve within a few weeks, but it is just as likely that it will not, or even that it will get worse. Tiredness is cumulative, and you don't get the weekend to catch up.

Men sometimes think they must be as tired as the woman because they are more tired than they have ever been before. Peter Walker, a postnatal teacher and father of two, says that under normal circumstances this is almost never true. 'I see men and women after birth. The women are either hyper, or they look absolutely drained and you see them staring into space. You don't get that with the men.'

If you catch yourself thinking she can't be as tired as all that, try being up all the time she is for a week, then double or even triple it for the cumulative effect of birth, breastfeeding and the last days, weeks or months.

> One night at about 10 o'clock when I had been walking our crying baby round and round the sitting room for at least an hour, my partner came up and said – 'I'm sorry but I have just GOT to go to bed.' And he went. I carried on walking, tears now running down my face as well, thinking – 'I suppose I haven't GOT to go to bed.' I was certainly more tired than he was since I was doing all the nights, but there I was and there was nothing I could do about it.
>
> It wasn't entirely his fault. I should have handed him the baby ages before and said I was going to bed. I just tended to hang on to my son when he was crying, and it hadn't

occurred to me that I would be deserted and left to do it without even a bit of company.

Jennifer, son 2 yrs

Sharing the load is clearly the best way to reduce individual tiredness and to keep some sort of balance in your need for sleep (and perhaps for sex). It may help if you regard your collective energy as a joint resource – though this requires very honest assessment.

If one of you is doing all the nights – for instance to breastfeed – that one should get a chance to sleep in or have an afternoon rest at weekends or whenever possible. It is important to reassess occasionally what each of you is doing. It is easy to get stuck in a rut. If you breastfeed, for example it quickly becomes established that the woman does the nights. She gets used to hearing the baby and he gets used to not hearing. Don't forget that once breastfeeding stops, dealing with night-waking can be shared.

I breastfed our son for nine months, so I did all the nights. Once I had stopped feeding, I still did all the nights. I was used to it, assumed the baby needed me, and my partner just didn't wake up. Then our son went through a patch of being awake for an hour or two in the night and I suddenly thought – this is ridiculous. Why am I doing it all? We talked it over and instituted alternate nights on duty. We should have done it much earlier.

Claire, son 2 yrs

When you first hand over some of the nights you will have to be ruthless about waking your partner. And when you first take over nights, you will need to go to sleep telling yourself you are listening for the baby. Do not rely on your partner to wake you up, or she will never get a genuinely undisturbed night.

It will help a lot if the father has always done some night duties so the baby is not unsettled by sometimes getting daddy instead of mummy at night. This also applies to the daytime. The child will, not unreasonably, turn first to whichever parent he spends most time with, so it is easy for both parents to fall into the trap of letting whoever does most do all. To avoid this, the primary carer needs to be prepared to stand back, and the less-present parent needs to be sure to stay in touch. Young children change by the day, and they are very conscious of who is around. If you are going to be involved in parenting, you do need to be with them on a fairly regular basis.

Sharing out the tiredness – and with it some of the worries of parenthood – should help keep your relationship (both general and sexual) on a more even keel. If you want sex and your partner is too tired, address the tiredness. Plan breaks and lie-ins – and if you promise one, stick to it!

Finding times to make love when you are not exhausted can be difficult, especially when a baby is very young and unpredictable. Once some kind of routine is established, which can be anything from six weeks to three years depending on your child and your determination, you should be able to work something in around daytime naps and bedtimes.

You may have to accept that by a certain time at night (ten, eleven, nine?) one or both of you is good for nothing but a cuddle and sleep. Having a cut-off time like this is a good way of reducing the number of advances and rejections and, when possible, of concentrating the mind on getting to bed earlier.

When you do get round to making love, be aware that tired people tend to be slower to get aroused and slower to reach orgasm. If you are going to make love with one or both of you very tired, you need to be realistic about how you do it and what you expect. This means talking very honestly about what you want and what you feel up to.

One of you may be happy to make love but not want to feel under pressure to reach orgasm, or you may want to orgasm, in which case the less-tired partner will need to be prepared to work a bit harder. There are less energetic ways of making love. Smaller movements are not necessarily less satisfying and there are positions that do not leave either of you balanced on a few muscles. Try both lying down and see what you can do (see Appendix B for ideas).

Whatever you do or don't do, it is crucial to have an understanding that saying no is saying no to the action and not to the person. There is no point in feeling rejected when the problem is simply exhaustion. Realism is vital. You will probably not be able to eradicate tiredness, at least in the first weeks or months of your child's life, but it is worth minimizing. As one parent put it, 'When you are well rested, everything is possible, when you are not, nothing is possible.'

Pain and Soreness

Some pain or discomfort during sex after birth is, unfortunately, quite common. One study found 20 per cent of women still had pain or discomfort during intercourse (known medically as dyspareunia) three months after the birth. A study looking only at first-time mothers put this figure as high as 40 per cent. This study found the number still suffering fell to 18 per cent at six months and 8 per cent at a year.

It is perhaps not surprising that the combination of childbirth and a relatively rapid return to sex causes problems for some people. But it seems unlikely that it is really necessary for this many people to suffer. Some of the solutions lie in changes in medical practice. We can try to influence these by asking the right questions and making the right demands, but ultimately we have to live with the practice of the day. Other solutions lie in some (often quite simple) pieces of advice that should be – but are not – routinely given to new parents. The rest of this chapter (and Chapter 9) attempts to fill some of the gaps.

Caesarean
The pain after a Caesarean will probably be greater than after most vaginal deliveries, and you may take a few weeks longer to start to feel reasonable again. During love-making you will need to keep his weight off the scar for the first three months or so. If you have significant pain after this – either generally, or during sex or orgasm – it is probably worth seeing a doctor, to check that you do not have a low-level infection that is causing the problem.

Some of the information that follows may not apply to you if your baby was born by Caesarean, but much of it will.

Dryness

One of the simplest and most common reasons for discomfort or soreness during intercourse after childbirth is dryness. This can be because the woman is simply not turned on enough to be ready for penetration, something that may be caused or exacerbated by anxiety, distraction (will the baby wake up?), tiredness, fear of another pregnancy, etc. and/or it can be due to hormonal changes interfering with your natural lubrication, which is especially likely if you are breastfeeding.

The answer to the first cause is longer or more appropriate foreplay. This may require some discussion, as both emotional and physical needs can be quite changed after a baby is born. Something relaxing – like a glass of wine – may also help. (More on possible psychological factors in Chapter 9.)

Dryness due to hormones – high levels of prolactin and low levels of oestrogen – is easily solved by using a water-based lubricant like KY Jelly. This is readily available from chemists and can be used to top up your natural lubrication until your body returns to normal after the birth or when you stop breastfeeding.

Do be sure that the lubricant is water-based, as oil-based products (like Vaseline) can irritate the vagina and damage condoms, diaphragms and caps.

I had eight stitches with my first child but had no pain (on intercourse) at all. We used LOTS of KY Jelly and built up to it slowly. My husband and I started having baths together within a week and gentle touching and petting and within three weeks we had sex without any pain. My husband was very understanding and gentle and let me make all the moves when I was ready. We always talked about how we felt and made allowances for tiredness.

Rashpal, sons 3 yrs and 1 yr

Lubrication was OK up to about six weeks, then it dipped off until she stopped breastfeeding. We didn't use KY Jelly. She had largely gone off sex and we felt that if her body wasn't

providing the lubrication then she wasn't ready. I don't like
KY Jelly. You can't tell what is going on, you are less aware of
the other person.

Lawrence, son 10 m

It is clearly very important that KY is not used to do something
one or both of you does not really want, or to penetrate too soon.
But, used sensitively, it can be very useful in regaining confidence
after the birth and in allowing you to return to making love comfortably when you want to.

Occasionally vaginal dryness can be extreme, making you
feel very sore all the time. This may be due to very low levels of
oestrogen.

After the birth of my first son, I was so sore down there I was
red raw. It took six months and three doctors before oestrogen
deficiency was diagnosed. One day my husband came home
and found me almost literally climbing the walls and said we
have got to do something about this. We had thought it was
an infection. We'd tried every cream under the sun, but it
wasn't an infection. After the second birth, we knew what
it was. I went straight on an oestrogen pill which cured it
immediately.

Jenny, sons 3 yrs and 1 yr

Extreme dryness due to oestrogen deficiency can be treated with
oestrogen cream or pills. The advantage of cream is that it goes
straight on to the affected area and so will not affect breastmilk.
Oestrogen taken by mouth will go through to a breastfed baby, but
research so far suggests that low doses of oestrogen do not do any
harm. This condition is not widely understood, so if your GP is not
sympathetic, try a Family Planning Clinic.

Anxiety

Pain during intercourse is often put down to anxiety. This can be
very upsetting if you are sure it has a different cause. Frequently, of

course, the anxiety is the result of the pain.

Occasionally, however, anxiety or tension is enough to cause pain during intercourse – it may make you feel too tight, or you may feel pain you cannot pinpoint to any particular place. Having an alcoholic drink may help (but men beware of becoming less sensitive to your partner's pain). Try whatever relaxes you.

> When we tried sex it was very painful, screaming agony, and this was until at least three to four months after the birth. I must have vaguely mentioned this to my parents who said I must get help. So when I went to the doctor for some other reason, when the baby was about four months, I asked him about it. He told me to try and make saliva during the sexual act. I suppose you need to be relaxed to do this. It worked!
>
> **Marion, daughter 3 yrs, son 1 yr**

If your relaxation technique, whatever it may be, does help, you will probably find that after a few pain-free sessions you won't need it any more. If it doesn't work, do not despair. Read on...

Pain During Intercourse

Pain during intercourse (known medically as dyspareunia) may be 'superficial' – that is, on the outside, around the perineum and the entrance to the vagina – or 'deep', meaning right up inside. Superficial in this context does NOT mean minimal or unimportant. Superficial pain can be excruciating and is the more common type of pain during intercourse after childbirth.

Superficial dyspareunia is most likely to be due to an episiotomy or tear. If you have had neither of these, it may come from bruising, grazing, or very small tears in the labia (lips around the vagina) that did not need stitching and may not even have been mentioned to you. The causes of deep dyspareunia, with no other symptoms, are less obvious but can be just as uncomfortable.

Pain during intercourse usually goes with time. At what stage you want to investigate further will depend on how you and your partner feel, and on what you think might be the matter.

Three months is often cited as a time when you might seek help if you are still having problems, but a great many cases of pain during intercourse do resolve themselves after three months. Some time between three months and six months might be a good time to have a think about what could be causing the problems, even if you decide to leave it a bit longer before you involve outsiders.

Infections need to be treated as soon as possible, so if your scar is very red or there is visible pus, you have smelly discharge or a fever, or if you just think you have an infection, do see a doctor.

Hard, unyielding scars that will not stretch properly may also need relatively early treatment. They will not get any worse, but obstetric physiotherapy is more likely to be successful before six months than after, although it is still worth trying even at a year (see Physiotherapy, below).

Notice how the pain changes over a period of time. If it is becoming less intense, then it will probably go away by itself in time. If it is as bad at six months as it was at six weeks, you may want to seek help now.

Some women are keen to seek medical help as soon as possible, but others may be reluctant. Women who have felt very acutely the prodding and poking – the invasion of their bodies – during pregnancy and childbirth may feel they cannot face yet more internal examinations, let alone the possibility that some form of treatment might be recommended.

You have been flat on your back with your legs in the air so many times. The last thing you are going to do – unless you are in constant excruciating pain – is go and knock on the doctor's door and say please can I get undressed and put my legs in the air and be examined AGAIN...Even when I knew things weren't right I put off going to the doctor because I just really didn't want to be examined again.

Ann, daughter 7 m

As her partner, you may be determined to get this problem sorted out – and you may be right – but you need to be very understanding about her fears. They are not unreasonable when you think what she has so recently been through. As one mother put it, 'No account is taken of the damage done inside your head.'

Talk about the problem between you. Use a mirror and have a look and a feel around to see if you can work out exactly where or what the problem is. Every problem is different and so is every couple. Each set of circumstances will lead to different decisions about what to do and when.

When my daughter was a few months old, I went to the doctor about something to do with her. Somehow it came out that my episiotomy still hurt and sex was not happening much. The doctor was very keen to talk about this. I think it was concern for my partner. I really had other things to worry about. I just wanted to sort out the problem I had gone in there for. Sex was not at the top of my list at that stage. My episiotomy scar went on hurting when we made love for over a year, but eventually it sorted itself out.

Tanya, daughter 3 yrs, son 4 m

After the twins were born I had quite a lot of pain. The doctor was very sympathetic but couldn't find anything. She said the stitching looked fine and it did. I think it was psychological. I just couldn't quite believe I would ever be OK again, and when you are all tensed up it does hurt.

After my third child I had less pain, but it felt and looked wrong. I went to the GP who was very nice and said it didn't look as though I had been stitched very well, and I ought to go back to the consultant. He was very off-hand and said, 'After three children what do you expect, just wait.' Because he was so brusque, I didn't trust him, and we thought if I did need restitching we wanted to do it as soon as possible. So I went privately for a second opinion. In fact the private consultant said exactly the same thing – but he said it nicely. He told us to just leave it and it would be OK in about nine months. And it was.

Lucy, twins 6 yrs, daughter 1 yr

After my son was born a junior doctor stitched me up. She kept saying, 'I don't know where this bit goes.' We didn't

have sex for six months. It hurt to sit down. I was too frightened to try having sex. I saw a specialist and he said there was
nothing wrong. When we did make love it was very uncomfortable. There was a lump. There was a point that hurt if it
was pressed, a ridge. I think I had been stitched too tight.
Eventually a specialist offered to recut and resew, but I didn't
fancy that. By being careful about positions, we managed. It
didn't affect sex too much once we got going. John used to
complain jokingly – I think jokingly – but he was generally
understanding.

It went on being uncomfortable for two and a half years,
until my second child was born. I had her at home and
insisted my GP sew me up very carefully. Now it feels fine.

Maura, son 2 yrs, daughter 3 m

Sex after my son was born was bloody painful. I went to several doctors. I was told there was skin caught. I could only
have sex in certain positions; on top was pure agony, side-by-
side was OK. Sex hurt until I finally had it redone two years
after the birth. I don't know why I didn't have it done before.
I suppose I hoped it would sort itself out.

Suzie, son 8 yrs

I had pain in my perineal scar [during sex] at six weeks and it
just continued. At about six months I had it checked by a
doctor who said it was oedema [swelling] around the scar
which would eventually settle by 11–12 months. And it did.

Lucia, children 3 yrs and 1 yr

Seeking Help

Some doctors are excellent, well informed and understanding.
Others are not. Many do not understand how much a woman may
loathe internal examinations nor how vulnerable she may be feeling in this period of early motherhood.

Leading midwifery researcher Jennifer Sleep says, 'GPs can be
quite dismissive [of pain during sex]: "A bottle of wine, a tube of

KY Jelly and lie back and think of England" – I've heard that more than once.'

A bottle of wine and a tube of KY might help a few people, but this kind of insensitivity does not. And it is, unfortunately, not limited to GPs.

> After about six months, we tried making love. Penetration was physically impossible. I had been stitched up incorrectly. I saw a gynaecologist who apart from giving me a set of glass dilators, also told me that, 'If you had been married to a man who had forced his way in, you'd be all right by now.' By this time I felt as if it was all my fault...I used the dilators alone (because my husband seemed to think this was something I should deal with) twice a day for two months. I had been told to find time alone, to be relaxed to use these things. I was working part-time, had a lively baby who was walking at eight and a half months and I was expected to find time to relax!
>
> **Cassie, daughter 2 yrs**

Sex therapists generally talk about trainers rather than dilators, and would usually use the warmer and perhaps less off-putting plastic variety rather than glass. It would also have helped if Cassie's doctor had suggested ways her partner could help – at the very least by taking the baby.

Health professionals rarely think of such things, however, so it is down to male partners to be there at the appointment and to think through how you can best help with any treatment that is recommended.

If your GP is unsympathetic, you can go to a Family Planning Clinic instead. They specialize in sexual matters and may even be better able to spot the problem than a GP who is by definition a generalist.

Sometimes – in fact, quite often – the doctor will say he or she can find nothing wrong. If you have been examined lying down, which is the usual way, suggest they examine you while you are standing up. Sometimes a bit of scar tissue that is inside or at the entrance to the vagina may be hard to feel lying down but will come to the surface when you are standing.

Being told 'there is nothing wrong' can be as much of a problem as being told there is something.

> At the six-week check I was asked if there were any problems [with sex] but you don't really know by then. When we did do it, sex was really painful on entering. It was OK once he was in, but we could only do it in certain positions and it didn't get any better. I went to my GP but she couldn't find anything. She said if I expected everything to be the same after having a baby I was mistaken, so I thought I just had to put up with it...I have quite an understanding husband, but in the end I shut up, because I thought he'd just think I was making excuses. It was a strain, though. When he said, 'Let's make love,' I thought 'Oh God.'
>
> Jeanette, son 1 yr

Being told 'there is nothing wrong' does NOT mean you are making a fuss about nothing. Nor does it mean that pain during intercourse is something you just have to put up with. It means either that there is a psychological element to the pain or (equally likely) that the person examining you has failed to find the physical cause.

Jeanette continues:

> Finally, when my son was about 13 months old, I found a loop of skin at the entrance to my vagina. I went back to the GP. She said 'well done' for finding it and told me I would have to go to the hospital. I had to be recut and resewn. I was very angry. But after the operation everything was fine. I couldn't believe what I had put up with for 13 months. Now at last I can lie back and relax.

If you think the doctor has missed something physical, try the Family Planning Clinic or ask to be referred – if necessary insist on being referred – to a specialist. If the pain is superficial ask for the nearest hospital Vulval Clinic or obstetric physiotherapist. Otherwise you need a consultant obstetrician/gynaecologist. If you are going as a private patient, you can choose your consultant. Ask around before you make an appointment. Local NCT groups, postnatal groups, health visitors, etc. may know which consultants are best for this sort of problem.

If you think your problem is psychological you could go straight to a good sex therapist (see Further Information). Do both remember that pain with a psychosomatic origin is just as real and painful as any other pain. Only the means of getting rid of it is different: talking and understanding (perhaps with professional guidance) rather than physical treatment.

When a medical examination does find a physical problem, you may be told to wait a few weeks or months to see if it improves. If something more drastic is suggested – like being recut and resewn – do not forget that it is still up to you what you do and when. You may want the operation as quickly as possible. On the other hand, you might want to ask to try physiotherapy before resorting to surgery or, if you are in any doubt about the doctor's diagnosis, you can seek a second opinion.

If you are planning another baby soon, you might consider leaving the resewing until after the next birth when you may have to be stitched anyway. This obviously depends on how well you would both cope in the mean time (see Coping with Lack of Sex, in Chapter 9).

It may be a relief to find a medical professional who recognizes and understands the problems you are having. It may also be upsetting if treatment is recommended. Partners – who are not suffering directly – will need to be very understanding. Any form of additional interference with this part of the body (which she may just be trying to reclaim as her own) can be quite upsetting, even if it is painless. Being told that she will need to be recut and resewn can be devastating. Imagine your own genitals had been cut or torn, stitched and painful and now you were asked to do it all again, and you shouldn't find it hard to be sympathetic.

Physiotherapy
Physiotherapy is sometimes used to treat painful sex after childbirth. It may just involve advice, massage and exercises, or it may use ultrasound or occasionally Pulsed Electromagnetic Energy (PEME) – both of which are painless.

ULTRASOUND

Ultrasound has been used with some success on wounds elsewhere in the body. It is thought to help when a wound has not healed properly, or when a scar has hardened and does not stretch as it should. If, for example, penetration is difficult and you feel it is because you have been stitched too tight, ultrasound may help soften the scar tissue so that it will stretch better. If you have a hard lump of scar that digs into you during sex, ultrasound may be able to soften it enough to allow you to make love without pain.

The physiotherapist may ask you to try making love soon after the treatment, to reinforce the additional stretchiness. Take it very gently, and if it hurts too much, stop.

There is little scientific understanding of the use of ultrasound on painful perineal scars, but it does seem to help some women.

> I had a tear and it was sore for quite a long time. At about three months I went to the doctor, but it wasn't until I had four private sessions with an obstetric physiotherapist that it started to get better. Now it is a lot better.
>
> Nicola, son 10 m

Her partner Laurance adds: 'We would never have known about the physio if I hadn't been a doctor. It was never mentioned by the GP.'

Not all doctors are very aware of the use of obstetric physiotherapy, so if you have trouble getting yourself referred, write to the Secretary of the Association of Chartered Physiotherapists in Obstetrics and Gynaecology, at the Chartered Society of Physiotherapists (see Further Information). They can advise you on how to get to a physiotherapist, either privately or on the NHS.

Coping with Painful Sex

If sex is painful you may simply want nothing to do with it until things improve. This is eminently reasonable and nobody who is finding sex uncomfortable should ever be pushed into doing it.

If, however, you very much want to make love and the single

barrier is one painful area, you may find you can work round it, at least to some extent. Try out different positions. Having the woman on top or lying side by side may take pressure off the perineum. Limiting penetration may help with deeper dyspareunia (*see Appendix B*).

If penetration is the problem, there are plenty of non-penetrative sexual acts. Various forms of mutual masturbation (not necessarily simultaneous) and oral sex may be satisfactory alternatives (*see Appendix B again*).

Whatever you try, take it gently, checking she is all right at each stage. Be very honest about pain and be prepared to abandon the whole thing at any point. The aim is to find a pleasurable way of making love, NOT to grin and bear it.

The Pelvic Floor Muscles

The pelvic floor muscles (which support the vagina and the urethra) can be quite lax after childbirth (*see Figure 1 and the section on Pelvic Floor Exercises in Chapter 2, page 19*). This affects general comfort, ability to retain urine (and, very occasionally, faeces) and quality of sex. All will improve with time and exercise.

A weak pelvic floor can make you feel heavy and achy around the vaginal and perineal area, and this may get worse when you have a period or after sex. Stress incontinence affects up to 50 per cent of women just after the birth and leaves you leaking urine when you cough, sneeze, etc. More rarely, it can also make you pee during sex (from pressure on the bladder) or when you orgasm.

Most stress incontinence should clear up by three to six months after the birth. In the meantime, tighten the pelvic floor and cross your legs before you cough – and pee before you make love!

How much you notice any sexual effect of a weak pelvic floor will depend on what you were used to before (and on how much you are doing it). Although it is possible to have perfectly satisfactory sex with a weak pelvic floor, you may find sex is better – for both of you – when the muscles are stronger.

Like any other muscle the pelvic floor can be strengthened with exercise. Research has found that both general exercise (swimming, dancing, yoga, postnatal exercises, walking, keep fit, etc.) and specific pelvic floor exercises are effective in strengthening the pelvic floor. Interestingly, women who take general exercise have been found to have stronger pelvic floors than those who ONLY do pelvic floor exercises. Not surprisingly, doing both is likely to get the best results.

Postnatal pelvic floor exercises are basically the same as those done during pregnancy (*see page 19*), but now you need to be careful not to overdo it. If the muscles start to ache or shiver, stop. Little and often is best.

You can test your pelvic floor strength in a number of ways (depending on how long it is since the birth): try stopping urine mid-flow (but don't do this too often); jump up and down and cough and see if you leak; try tightening the muscles while you are making love – can you and/or your partner feel a difference?

If you are getting very severe aching or if exercises do not seem to help, ask to see a physiotherapist. She will design a programme of exercise specific to you and help you assess your progress. She might also use a machine giving neurotrophic stimulation (also called eurotrophic stimulation) or interferential therapy. These are both intended to stimulate the muscle. They may feel a bit like pins and needles but should never hurt. Nobody knows if these treatments are really more helpful than exercises alone, but used properly they do not seem to do any harm.

If you were not aware of your pelvic floor muscles before pregnancy and birth, you may find your new awareness and strength gives you a pleasant surprise if you try using them during sex.

I didn't know pelvic floor muscles existed until I got pregnant and was told to do exercises with them. After the birth they were very weak and achy and I had to do more exercises and go for physiotherapy. Now they are much stronger and I am also aware of them in a way I never was before. If I tighten them when we're making love – or alternate tightening and releasing – it can increase the sensation for me and, I think, for my partner. Something good for sex that has come out of childbirth!

Chrissie, son 2 yrs

Haemorrhoids

Haemorrhoids are a very common and little talked about side-effect of pregnancy and childbirth. They may appear during pregnancy and be exacerbated by the birth, or they may appear as a result of the birth. Women are often told that haemorrhoids will go in a few weeks. Sometimes they do. Sometimes they don't. But they do improve.

There is no proven way of completely ridding yourself of long-term haemorrhoids. Some people say a clove of garlic put just inside the anus and replaced whenever it comes out can substantially shrink them.

Otherwise it is a matter of controlling them with lubricant, creams, pushing them back into place and (perhaps most of all) not getting constipated.

There are operations available to remove haemorrhoids but these should be an absolute last resort. They should always be left until you have finished having children, and one very senior physiotherapist went so far as to say that such operations can do more harm than good.

Orgasm

While some women find orgasm is better after childbirth, others find it more difficult. If there is no obvious reason (like soreness), this is most likely to be due to tiredness and distraction, and should be temporary.

A few women say that problems with orgasm persist. There appears to be no scientific research on this so there may be causes we do not know about. It may simply be that the responsibilities of parenthood are making it difficult to relax completely and let go while making love.

Fran Reader, a gynaecologist and sex therapist, has a theory about a possible physical cause in women who were previously able to orgasm through penetrative sex alone. Only a minority of women are ever able to do this and it comes from a very close fit around the penis that leads to indirect tugging on the labia minora, which in turn stimulates the clitoris. If after childbirth the shape of the vaginal opening and the labia are slightly changed, this particular fit may no longer exist.

In the short term, changing positions to get more clitoral stimulation may help (*see Appendix B*). This can be done either directly or by having the woman on top leaning forward so that the clitoris is more affected by the movements of intercourse.

In the longer term, strengthening the pelvic floor muscles may allow you to recreate something like the original fit (or perhaps even create it for the first time!).

9

PSYCHOLOGICAL HURDLES

Whatever your physical problems, they can be exacerbated, or even caused, by psychological problems – and vice versa. Mind and body are extremely closely linked, especially when it comes to sex.

By 'psychological problems' I do not necessarily mean anything very dramatic – just feelings, thoughts, preoccupations that can affect or interfere with your life and relationships.

The period after a baby is born is very intense. There are few things as emotionally powerful as the birth of your own child, and few things that change your life and priorities as quickly or as completely.

There is bound to be a certain amount of rethinking to be done – and a certain amount of reshaping of relationships. Some people adapt very easily to parenthood. Others find it harder. And it does not necessarily have anything to do with how much the baby is wanted. It may be more a matter of how much your lifestyle and your relationship are being asked to change.

It is not at all uncommon for life to change dramatically and for the relationship to take months or even a year or two to catch up. In the mean time there may be resentment, misunderstandings and regular harsh words. The woman may resent her partner who does not have to feed the baby at 3 a.m., does not have sore genitals and in the early months at least is probably the only one who escapes each day to a workplace where he can go to the loo on his own. The man may be feeling left out and ignored and be unable to understand why his partner is foul to him if he is so much as 10 minutes late in from work. Sex may be completely off the menu or causing constant tension between you. If this is you, take heart.

The same sort of thing is happening in hundreds, if not thousands, of other new families and it will not go on for ever.

If you look at how often this sort of scenario occurs, it can only be described as 'normal', though it clearly cannot be allowed to go on for too long. Recognize it now and it should be possible to create a more amicable arrangement.

Talk about your feelings, in as blame-free a way as possible. This may not be easy – especially if direct communication has not been a feature of your relationship so far. But it is the only way to sort out problems relatively quickly and fairly. Leaving things for too long allows resentment to build up into a real wall between you, and that makes it even harder to talk.

Be prepared to make some changes – if necessary, reverse decisions made before the baby was born. This is a time of change, of adapting and adjusting to what has just happened and to what the future holds. Nothing will be solved overnight (though it may start to be) but it will happen a lot more quickly if everything is brought out into the open.

The rest of this chapter looks at some of the causes of 'marital' and sexual unhappiness in the postnatal period. In almost every case – from birth trauma to changed roles in the household – the answer starts with recognizing, admitting and trying to understand the problem from both your points of view. Men and women are different and parenthood often exacerbates these differences, highlighting the weakest as well as the strongest points in your relationship.

Some couples communicate quite naturally. For others it is a real struggle. Some men in particular may never have talked about their feelings before. They will need to make a real effort, and their partners will have to be quite patient. If you do want to improve your relationship, however, now is the time to start talking and listening.

Effects of the Birth

The emotional condition in which you begin your lives as parents is partly dependent on the birth. So is your starting point for a return to your sex life. Birth is a sexual event. Not that it feels remotely like it (nobody I have met has ever thought so). But, at its best, childbirth can be an intensely intimate experience between you and your partner, and it is undeniably the biological culmination of your sexual relationship.

It is not surprising then that how the birth goes, emotionally as well as physically, can affect your sexuality. The effect can be positive or negative, though the positive tends to be first on the relationship and only later on sex itself.

We have already looked at some reactions to birth in the chapters on Fathers at the Birth (see *page 41*) and The Early Days (*see page 69*). A few days or even weeks of feeling a bit shocked or off-balance (especially for women) is not unusual. If you can talk it over, the shock and the memory usually fade and all is well.

> I was absolutely traumatized by the first birth. I was at home, which was where I wanted to be, my partner was great, the midwife was fine, but the pain was staggering, I hated tearing and being stitched and the whole thing left me in a state of shock. I couldn't imagine how my mother had done this FIVE times. I now have four children. The oldest is five.
>
> **Susan, four children 5 yrs, 4 yrs, 2 yrs and 8 m**

Susan recovered quickly and was never as shocked again. Her husband, David, was very moved by all four births. In fact, he says, they more or less filled the emotional gap left by a lack of sex in six years of pregnancy, breastfeeding and quick conception.

> We have been very lucky to have had four very good birth experiences. Being in your own bed together with this tiny newborn is more intense and intimate than sex can ever be. It makes sex as an emotional event seem almost a let-down.

A birth does not have to be quick or easy to be a positive experience. Some couples can go through a long labour and an emergency Caesarean and still come out feeling good about the whole thing.

> It was all quite dramatic. They suddenly said the baby was stuck and everything started to move very fast. But they took

us with them all the time. Everything was explained, and we never doubted that they were doing the right thing.

Harriet, son 1 yr

Harriet recovered more quickly than many people do after 'natural' births. It is not so much what actually happens that matters as how you feel about it: your expectations, and how you were treated. Any feeling of failure or mistreatment makes the trauma much more difficult to deal with.

> After all the preparation in antenatal classes and everything, I ended up having an emergency Caesarean. I feel it was due to shortage of staff. I feel it was unnecessary. There was a ward full of Caesareans.
>
> I was 17 days overdue so they started inducing me. Then they stopped inducing me because it got too busy. When I went down to the delivery suite the monitoring machine was not working properly. In the labour room there were three changes of staff all voicing different opinions about what was happening with me.
>
> At one point a doctor was talking to my partner and suddenly shoved a needle in my hand. He didn't even tell me. I didn't even know he was there. It was like an assault.
>
> The doctors kept doing internals. All these men going up my fanny every five minutes. I just wanted somebody to get them to go away. They kept taking blood from the baby's head and kept getting useless results and doing it all again. Another internal, another blood sample from the baby. Eventually the baby went into distress – not surprising really.
>
> I felt really violated. Now I feel my body isn't mine any more. All those internals have changed the way I feel about sex – and I didn't even have a vaginal delivery.

Janine, daughter 4 m

Janine describes herself as feeling 'violated' and 'assaulted'. Other women use words like 'invaded' and even 'raped'. Research by one (female) GP found that some women had all the symptoms of Post

116

Traumatic Stress Disorder after rough internal examinations or forceps deliveries.

A birth with greater intervention is more likely to cause this sort of reaction, but a medically normal birth can still leave the couple traumatized if it is mishandled. Mary's son was eventually born 'normally', but hospital staff ignored her, sent her home after refusing to examine her (when she was several centimetres dilated and in great pain), tried to frighten her into unnecessary interventions and carried out some procedures without warning. Mary was left feeling bullied and abused. This also affected her partner, who felt he had failed her by being unable to prevent what was happening:

> I had no sexual drive for at least three months after the birth. I had to work things over in my mind; the pain and the birth. That certainly had an effect on me. You are not in control. You don't know what is going on. Perhaps I should have been better prepared. For three months it was very much on my mind. Then our son began to be his own person – more and more removed from his birth – and it wore off.

Both men and women can be affected by feelings of powerlessness and failure, particularly when the birth takes place in a large hospital. Men have often been brought up to protect the 'gentler sex', and to find themselves unable to do so can feel like an assault on their masculinity.

Equally, a woman may feel a failure for not giving birth 'naturally', for 'giving in' to an epidural or having to have a Caesarean. Needless to say, you are no less of a man or woman for being unable to control nature or hospital procedure. It is a great achievement to give birth or be part of a birth, however it goes. You may even have coped with MORE than someone who gave birth 'naturally'. But these feelings are real and can affect your attitude to sex and to each other. Your feelings need to be accepted and understood before they can be dismissed.

This is true of all the emotional traumas of birth. The more they can be talked about – and listened to in an understanding way – the easier they are to put away in your mind. Talk to each other, to friends who have had babies and to any relevant support groups (*see Further Information*). If this is not enough, see a counsellor or, if your problems are having a direct effect on your sex life, a sex therapist.

Upset or depression relating to the birth can come in a delayed reaction. Ann Dally, a counsellor for Birth Crisis, says women often come to her around five or six months after the birth, having just realized how traumatized they felt and feel.

Sex therapists sometimes find that when a couple comes to them with pain during intercourse (dyspareunia) for which no physical cause can be found, or with long-term fear of or loss of interest in sex, there is an unresolved birth trauma somewhere in the background. Just as some people are left with physical scars from birth, these people have a psychological wound. This is especially common where the traumas of birth have reawakened memories of sexual abuse, but it can also happen without any previous sexual trauma.

Denise Knowles, a counsellor for Relate, says there is also sometimes a subconscious connection made between penetration and pain. To put it very simplistically: penetrative sex led to pregnancy which led to labour and birth and pain. Therefore, penetration produces pain. This can affect either the woman who suffered the pain, or the man who watched her go through it and felt that he was (at least in part) responsible.

Such a subconscious connection, or fear of another pregnancy, can result in psychosomatic pain on her part or in either partner going off sex, even very occasionally to the point of impotence.

If you feel that any of these problems apply to you, do speak up. Even men like John (in Chapter 4, on Fathers at the Birth), who found himself impotent towards his wife after seeing her genitals during the birth, can be helped. Once again the beginning of the answer is to recognize the problem. If your traumas or fears have been causing serious physical symptoms (pain, impotence), you may need considerable time and care, or the help of a sex therapist to restore your sexual confidence.

A word of encouragement: the first birth is usually the hardest. And the fact that you had a difficult first birth (whether physically or psychologically) does not mean you will necessarily have trouble the second time. The last word to Laura on her three births:

My first birth was an incredible shock. It was in a very modern hospital. On arrival, I had my waters broken and a foetal scalp monitor attached. After four hours of very fierce painful contractions I moved across the room to the gas and air machine (an almost impossible feat). I then lost control completely, and the gas and air made it worse – the room swirled around me and I decided an epidural was the only option. I was in such agony. The epidural slowed down the labour and eventually led to a forceps delivery. That night I had to be catheterized [a tube into the urethra] in order to wee. I had excruciating piles and many stitches and could hardly walk even five days after the birth. We didn't try having sex until our daughter was six months old, and I was still sore. Every time I closed my eyes I was back in the delivery room and I could see the midwives and doctors standing round me on the delivery table as they had been during the forceps delivery. The birth really knocked the stuffing out of me. For about a year I was very nervous and had occasional panic attacks. At this time I felt I would never be able to face having another baby, which saddened me because I had never wanted an only child.

When our daughter was two, I began to feel ready to contemplate another pregnancy. I remained pessimistic about the birth, but in the event I had a very long but quite comfortable natural birth. I needed no pain relief and the whole thing left me feeling totally exhilarated. I felt I had climbed a great mountain and was standing at the summit – marvellous. Our son's birth led to really positive feelings about my body. My husband had also seemed very proud and impressed by the birth. I felt good about myself and that I was beautiful in his eyes. I began to feel sexy again, even from the moment of birth.

Our third child was born at home. It was as well that we had planned it that way because his birth was so quick we would never have got to hospital anyway. We were watching television at about 10.15 p.m. when I started to feel restless and uncomfortable sitting down. I went upstairs to bed and had a 'real' fierce contraction. Then three more. I struggled to the landing and called my husband. The baby was born about 45 minutes later in the bathroom, delivered by my husband, as the midwife didn't arrive until five minutes later. I felt calm and in control throughout and the children slept through the whole thing.

After such a positive birth experience, sexual feelings returned quite quickly and we first made love perhaps four weeks after the birth. There was no pain and much pleasure.

Laura, daughter 8 yrs, sons 5 yrs and 18 m

Body Image

Some men and women find that their view of the woman's body is changed by pregnancy and birth. Along with all her other problems, Mary felt this acutely.

Seeing your body function to reproduce is quite different from the sexual image. I find it quite alien. I think probably our society has got that a bit skewed.

Most of us are not brought up with birth going on around us, and the dominant image of the body in most of the media is both misleading (careful lighting, layers of make-up, hair sprays and wind machines) and very much the individual/sexual rather than the familial/reproductive. David again:

In primitive cultures sex is closely linked with motherhood and family. Here it is split. It is sex first and only secondly you can have children. Then thirdly there is sex again.

This makes for an image of the female body that is slim, firm and unflabby, breasts big enough but not too big, skin clear, eyes bright. All rather unrealistic in the months – or even years – after a baby is born. Bellies take a while to go down, and stretch marks to fade (they do not go away completely). Weight gained in pregnancy may not immediately fall off, and you won't be getting much beauty sleep.

Try not to expect too much of yourself, or of her. The female body does adapt again to not being pregnant and will return to looking similar to before (and sometimes 'better'), but it may take time. Breasts will remain large while you are breastfeeding, then shrink when the baby is weaned. They do not always go back to exactly what they were before you were pregnant – they may remain a little larger or get a little smaller.

Breastfeeding helps the body to return to normal internally and some women find that it also helps take the extra weight off. Others are not able to lose weight until the baby is weaned. And the period of breastfeeding is certainly not a time for restrictive diets.

Try not to allow yourselves to be hoodwinked by the media, or by new mother friends who have made an effort because you are visiting. Most new mothers do not look like the ones in the adverts – who almost certainly are not new mothers!

You do not have to have jumped from the pages of *Playboy* to be a good lover. Jane Hawksley, Relate counsellor and sex therapist, says if you (or your partner) are feeling very unattractive, don't force yourselves to make love under 100-watt bulbs. Dim the lights and try to concentrate on the less visual aspects of love-making.

Women often worry unduly about their men's reactions to a bit of extra fat or wrinkles. You may find he is not nearly as concerned as you think.

My wife worries I might have gone off her. Her body is changed by two children. She is not physically the same as when we met. I thought my view of her body might be affected by the physical changes during and after the births, but it hasn't been. She is much more concerned than me. Women think men will go off and look for a young 20-year-old body. But that doesn't appeal to me. I don't find my wife less attractive, if anything I find her more so.

Ray, daughters 4 yrs and 3 yrs

Some women who talk of their 'body image' interfering with sex do not mean the body as a whole, but the place where the baby came out. This may be the Caesarean scar, or the genital area.

Scars do fade (though of course they do not disappear) and genitals that look or feel misshapen should reshape as the muscles regain their strength with time and exercise.

Some people see scars and minor changes as the honourable badge of motherhood, or are simply unconcerned.

> I had never examined my perineum very closely before I had a baby, but I think my perineum is now about half the length it used to be, and the back wall of the vagina can bulge a little bit if my muscles are tired or the area is slightly full after love-making. But this causes me no trouble and any changed appearance has never bothered me or my partner. With a bit of luck it might make me less likely to tear with the next birth.
>
> **Chrissie, son 2 yrs**

Sometimes, however, women talk of feeling 'damaged' or 'mutilated'. Very occasionally, the vaginal or perineal area has real physical distortions as a result of a devastating birth or incompetent repair, but it is more often a matter of coming to terms with minor changes. In the case of the genitals – which are not easily seen – the mental image of what has happened may be far worse than the reality.

With both Caesarean scars and genital problems, try not to run shy of the area. Once any wounds are fully healed, touching and looking (with a mirror if necessary) should give you a more realistic idea of what has happened and help you (both) come to terms with it. Talk through how you feel. Men may also need to touch and look, especially with a Caesarean scar.

Sometimes women can be reluctant to make love for fear of exposing their bodies to their partners. So, if as her partner you are not put off by any changes in her appearance (or indeed haven't noticed any), do say something encouraging. A compliment at the right moment from the right person can work wonders.

...And Then There Were Three

You are a family. No longer just a couple, a purely one-to-one relationship. There are three (or more) of you now. There is no point in pretending otherwise; having a baby changes your relationship.

Perhaps you used to have control of your lives, freedom, time to spend together, and a spontaneous sex life. Now a little human, who cannot even walk, is in the driving seat 24 hours a day. You are more likely to find a milk-soaked sheet, a nappy or a jangly toy when you get into bed than the sexy body of your partner waiting to welcome you. The emotional and sexual landscape has changed.

In the early weeks and months, the needs of the baby are primary – and this is as it should be. The mother, in particular, is likely to be very wrapped up in the child. The effect of a new baby on its mother can be overwhelming. Some women find the love, responsibility and sheer emotion they feel when they look at their baby almost frighteningly powerful.

> When I was pregnant I was very shocked to hear a friend say, in a very matter-of-fact way and in front of her husband, that her baby son was now more important to her than her husband. But from the moment my son was born, he was more important than anyone or anything else – including my partner and myself. This made me feel painfully vulnerable. Suddenly all my life, all my happiness depended on this fragile little being.
>
> **Jennifer, son 2 yrs**

The vast majority of women find themselves giving and giving to the baby with nothing much left over.

> I get occasional guilt trips. I am devoting so much time and energy to the baby and I can't even find 20 minutes to give to my partner. It just doesn't seem to come from the same well of energy.
>
> **Emma, daughter 4 m**

Biologically, of course, this all makes perfect sense – the next generation is more important than the last one – but that doesn't necessarily make it any easier. Some fathers will feel as involved with the baby as the mother, or almost so; perhaps especially if they have been at the birth and are at home for a while afterwards. Other men may feel quite excluded and replaced.

If as a father you are feeling put out, remember that your partner almost certainly doesn't love you any less (she may even love you more). The love for the baby is additional. Also, most women who put the baby before you also put the baby before themselves, so your position relative to her is unchanged.

This applies to allocation of time and attention, too. Try not to compare yourself with the baby in terms of your partner's attention – this is clearly unrealistic. Compare instead with the amount of time and attention she is giving herself (or indeed he is giving himself). The fact is that in the first months of a baby's life, adult needs – including sex – simply are not top priority.

It is quite possible that both partners may feel hard done by in the months after birth, though in different ways. He may feel pushed out of the intense mother–baby relationship, while she feels unsupported in her new, emotionally and physically draining role. Penny Mansfield of the marriage and partnership research group One Plus One found in her research that men often said they felt their partners didn't need them, whilst the women reacted to this with incredulity, saying they had never needed them so much in their lives.

In pregnancy everything was you (and especially the mother). Now everything is the baby. Relatives, health professionals, advice books are all focused on the baby now. And perhaps you are both putting all your affection into the baby as well.

The focus shifts from you to the baby. Suddenly both your cuddles are going into the baby. There's no one left to treat you as a baby. You both need to be mothered too. I had just had a baby and a major shift of identity – I wanted him to reassure me, and no doubt he wanted me to tell him he was still wonderful too.

Clemmie, daughter 9 m

New parents often feel in need of nurturing themselves – a need perhaps once met by the extended family and local community. Sometimes the grandparents still fill this role, but nowadays they are just as likely to be unavailable or inappropriate. Couples today are much more dependent on one another, so do try and give each other at least a cuddle and a word of reassurance now and then.

Modern relationships may be particularly vulnerable to the changes brought by a baby. Marriage used to be a matter of status and practicality. It was the only legitimate form of sexual relationship, closely linking sex and reproduction. It had clearly defined primary roles for men and women, and was designed to accommodate children.

Now the link between marriage and sex, and the link between sex and reproduction, are broken. You may have been sexually active for many years before marriage or childbirth. Couples expect a relationship to be a partnership of equals – and 'equal' is frequently confused with 'the same' or 'similar'. Modern 'committed' relationships are based on romantic love and the desire for, and expectation of, intimacy (usually including a reasonable sex life) and companionship.

Clearly the modern relationship requires much more realignment to accept a third party, especially one as emotionally and physically demanding as a baby. And the more similar your roles and day-to-day lives were before the baby, and the more your relationship was based round this 'equality', the more disrupted your relationship is likely to feel.

There is nothing that highlights the differences between the sexes more than becoming parents. Biologically, this is blindingly obvious, but many couples manage to minimize the impact through pregnancy, insisting that they will be equal parents once the baby is born. Many say this even when their practical arrangements (like who is at home and who is out earning) make this, to say the least, unlikely.

The present generation of new parents seems to have a real problem with the difference between what they say and what they do, according to Penny Mansfield, whose research has included extensive interviews with couples at the time of marriage and six years later. Ideology and expectation are way ahead of reality.

Couples talk a lot about sharing equally the care of the baby, domestic tasks, money earning, etc., but in practice many end up with something quite close to the old stereotypes. There is nothing wrong with the stereotypical pattern of wife and mother at home and husband and father as breadwinner, if it suits you. The important thing is to be sure your assumptions are not wildly different from your partner's and that you do not pretend one thing is happening when the reality is quite different. It is vital to be honest with yourselves and each other.

It is remarkable how dramatically, and often silently, assumptions can change when a baby is born. The most obvious (though by no means the only) example is the man who never expected his partner to do all the cooking or cleaning while they were both in full-time employment, but who suddenly expects her to do all things domestic now that she is at home with a baby. She, on the other hand, may feel she gave up work to look after the baby, not to spend all day hunched over the hoover or the stove. She may anyway be finding just caring for the baby quite hard enough without doing everything else as well. Assumptions and dishonesty (however unintended) can quickly lead to resentment, so do try and be open about both expectations and reality.

You may also be shocked by how differently you react to the baby. Perhaps because the woman has carried the baby inside her for nine months and then given birth, she is likely to react more immediately and undergo a quicker and more intense shift into motherhood. Men may take months to adjust to the fact of fatherhood, and what this means in day-to-day life.

This difference in adaptation can cause problems, especially if you have always understood each other easily in the past. You may feel that the baby has made you into strangers. It needn't, but you do have to accept that parenthood affects different sexes and different people differently. You may have to respect each other's individuality and try to treat your differing reactions as interesting rather than threatening. Unless your relationship is very young, it must have faced change before. This is a new, admittedly sizable, challenge.

You will need to talk (*see Communicating with Your Partner, page 153*) and may find that constant small changes (and perhaps a few big ones) are required over a period of time. Good relationships are not static, and at times of adaptation like this, change is sometimes needed just to stay still. (You can balance a stick on your finger only if you are constantly moving.)

You may find you fit comfortably into the traditional family pattern, and are happy with your separate and different (and NOT necessarily unequal) roles. Some people discover that this is what they have been waiting for.

For those not comfortable with the traditional arrangements, one key to survival is solidarity. The more you can share responsibility and decision-making, the less likely you are to have serious problems. If the problems of broken nights, worries about the baby's health, emotional attachment, clothes covered in puke, etc. are OUR problems; and if the adult problems of money, no time, no sex, a chaotic house, etc. are all OUR problems too; if WE can moan about it all TOGETHER – without it being one or the other's fault – life will be very much easier.

As ever, it is easy enough to say, but if you can manage an occasional laugh at the whole damn mess, all the better. A few books are listed in the Further Information chapter to help you to a giggle – and remind you that many other couples have been down this road before you, and most have survived.

While your relationship has been undergoing such changes, what has been happening in your sex life? Not a lot, quite probably. And the harder the adaptation of the relationship has been, the more true this is likely to be. The two, after all, are intimately linked.

There is no point in fighting the early stage of parenting. Feeling anxious, inadequate or guilty about lack of adult time and sex is only likely to extend sexual difficulties. Seeking gratification (be it intellectual, social or sexual) elsewhere is also likely to be counterproductive. If you cut yourself off from your partner now, you will have much more trouble returning. Put the baby and parenthood first. If necessary, survive on little or no sex for a while (*see Coping with Lack of Sex, page 156*) and try to create a solid base for the future. This state of affairs IS temporary.

Reclaiming Your Adult Relationship

There does come a point when you need to start to reclaim your adult relationship. And if it does not happen naturally, you may have to make a few conscious moves towards it. You clearly cannot go on for ever ignoring your own, and each other's needs – sexual or otherwise.

Family therapist Robin Skynner, in the book he wrote with John Cleese, *Families and How to Survive Them*, says reclaiming should happen alongside the child's 'toddler phase' – that is, when the child starts to explore the world outside his mother (or primary carer) and to begin to understand that he is a separate human being.

Looking at the most common family set-up where the mother is primary carer, Robin Skynner says that at this point the father needs to step forward for everyone's benefit. The baby needs a halfway house between mother and the outside world, the mother needs someone to fall back on as the closeness with the baby decreases, and the father is now in a position to 'reclaim his place as husband and lover, rather than just father'.

Be realistic. We are not talking about a sudden return to pre-baby living, but about making some time for yourselves as adults and gradually reclaiming your couple identity – and sex life. When this starts, how fast it progresses, and indeed whether you need to do it consciously at all, will depend on all three (or more) of you.

To feel like an adult, you have to be in touch with the adult world. So if one of you has been at home full-time, this is the moment to start getting out without the baby. If you find this daunting, take it gradually and gently.

After the first six months I started working part-time and that helped in terms of giving some space, some sense of myself as being separate...But we didn't go out (as a couple) for about a year, and then there was that feeling of we must rush back in case something has happened. That anxiety doesn't make for a good night out – and it's especially bad when you are still feeding. A couple of times we just threw in the hat and went home. We were more relaxed after the second baby. We knew that his every squeak did not have to be met with breastfeeding and we could pat his back and put him down, so he learned to go to sleep by himself.

The first time I was so wrapped up and absorbed in the baby. He was absolutely the most wonderful thing in my life. It's like when you learn to drive. At first all I could see was the car in front. As I got more confident, my field of vision widened to see husband/lover, work, etc. I feel that it is still widening out.

Janet, sons 8 yrs and 4 yrs

This process of widening horizons often continues until the youngest child goes to school. Indeed, research confirms that the preschool years are the hardest on the parents' relationship – at least until you get to the teens.

To begin giving the 'absorbed' mother some time away, it is often easiest for the father to take over for a while. Whether one of you is homebound or not, however, you do also need to get out together. So, if you haven't got one already, you now need a trusted babysitter (or two). Get out to a film, the theatre, the pub, dinner, a walk by the river, to friends (without the baby) – whatever you like to do as a couple.

The partner least in need of these outings may need to be the one to organize them. Some women, in particular, need a lot of help separating from the baby and returning to the adult relationship. If she is also expected to make all the necessary arrangements, it simply won't happen. Discuss what you want to do and who could babysit, then the man (or whoever is least baby-bound) get on and organize it.

Obviously, if you go out and one or both of you is really miserable all evening, forget it and try again later. It is more likely, however, that if you have a trusted person to babysit and you have left a phone number, once you are out of the house the feeling will be at least as much of liberation as concern.

Try to organize ahead so that you get a regular outing – once a month, once a week, whatever you want and can manage. You can also start to try and get some time to yourselves at home. This may mean trying to sort out your child's bedtime (or lack of it) or just allocating time away from the domestic grind.

You may need to make appointments – as you would if you were going out. Get a takeaway and a bottle of wine, sit together and watch telly or a video, read, talk, or just go to bed. Sexual spontaneity – in case you hadn't noticed – is a thing of the past. If you want to have time to make love at leisure, you will almost certainly have to plan for it. And perhaps use some unconventional times as well. Spontaneity may be part of the image of good sex, but it is not essential. Planned sex can be just as good. You might even enjoy the anticipation.

The more baby-bound partner may need time to separate herself (or himself) from the parental role before being ready to make love. The less baby-bound partner may find it helpful if once in a while he takes over on the domestic front, giving her time to be by herself, perhaps to have a bath, relax and remember her adult self. It helps if this is not ONLY done in relation to sex!

When you do want to make love, it may be useful to decide beforehand who is going to break off and get up if the baby wakes or cries. It is often a good idea if this is whichever of you is least distracted from sex by thoughts of the baby – usually the father. This allows the mother to let go and concentrate on making love. However, she needs to be confident that he really will listen, and that he will break off from sex and do something about it if the baby does wake. Otherwise she will not let go of her parenting role, whatever has been said.

If your attempts to reclaim your sexual relationship are floundering, take a look at the sections below on Coping with Lack of Sex and Returning to Sex. If there is something obviously interfering like a sick child, pain during intercourse, or extreme tiredness, give yourselves time. Have a look at relevant sections of this book and any others, or seek outside help. Address these issues before attempting to reclaim an adult 'normality' again. It is no good pushing yourselves into something that isn't working.

Do not feel guilty about giving yourselves and your relationship some time and attention. Your happiness is vital to your children as well as to you and, as Christopher Clulow (Director of the Tavistock Institute of Marital Studies) points out, children should not have to meet their parents' emotional needs as well as their own. He says, 'If children are not be burdened, the needs of parents must also be separately attended to in adult partnerships.'

Whilst children obviously need a lot of direct care and attention, they also need a comfortable atmosphere around them. Even babies pick up tension. Recent research found a link between parental stress – including dissatisfaction with the sexual relationship – and colic in babies. And older children are more consciously aware of whether their home is secure.

Finally, be realistic – about parenthood, partnership and sex. Life as a parent is one of carefully assessed compromise. You need balance – but it may be balance over days or months rather than hours, and the way it is achieved will keep changing, as your needs, and particularly the needs of your growing child, change.

Libby Purves, in her book *How Not to Be a Perfect Mother*, sums up the parenthood compromise neatly. She says, 'I am a mother and I would lay down my life for my children; but I see no reason to do it every single day.'

Partnership – even once 'reclaimed' – is likely to get less attention than before, and sex will probably be less frequent. This can have a positive effect, however. If something has a little rarity value you may find you put more effort into it and it is actually better.

Breastfeeding

The more relaxed you are about sexuality in general, the less likely you are to have serious problems with the psychological aspects of breastfeeding. Breasts are, of course, part of the sexual-reproductive system, so it is hardly surprising that breastfeeding can affect your sexuality. Both scientific research and anecdote suggest that breastfeeding can have a negative, positive or negligible effect on sex, depending entirely on the individuals concerned.

Effects on the Mother

As with pregnancy, breastfeeding may make you feel sexier, less sexy, or much the same. Any of these is normal, although a lowered level of sexual activity seems to be more common than a heightened one.

Many women – perhaps even most women, once feeding is established – find breastfeeding pleasurable. A few find it boosts their sexuality. Laura felt this after her third child was born:

> I really enjoyed my return to breastfeeding. I felt the breast-feeding enhanced my sexuality. We didn't mind making love with a replete baby sleeping peacefully beside us. It seemed appropriate somehow. If he stirred I would sometimes just move over and feed him – it seemed so natural.

Very occasionally, a woman may find breastfeeding itself sexually arousing. Laura recalls one – rare – occasion on which this happened:

> I was feeding my son one afternoon in a blissful semi-somnolent state when I became aware that I had become aroused almost – but not quite – to the point of orgasm. At other times of blissful relaxation while feeding I found my thoughts straying towards my husband and how nice it would be to have a cuddle. Maybe my libido is naturally higher at this time of day. What a pity that during this time when my babies have always slept peacefully society should require my husband to be at work!

Anyone who has involved the breasts in love-making knows that there is a connection between the breasts and the genitals and uterus. So it should not be surprising that breastfeeding can sometimes trigger a sexual response in the vagina and clitoris. There is absolutely nothing wrong with this. It is a natural functioning of the same hormonal pathway that causes afterpains (weakened labour-like contractions of the uterus) during breastfeeding soon after the birth. If you get sexual pleasure from breastfeeding, don't feel guilty – enjoy it.

Even for women who do not find breastfeeding sexually arousing, there can be powerful feelings of love and a sensuousness in the closeness to the baby. Once again this can cause feelings of guilt. Try not to let it. Feeling physically good with your baby is entirely natural and good for you both.

Breastfeeding can be, and usually is, enjoyed on a completely non-sexual level, though a few women do not enjoy it at all. Research suggests Laura is in a minority, it being more common for women to find their sexuality suppressed during the period of breastfeeding. As one mother put it, 'I found breastfeeding a total libido killer. I would rather have a cup of tea – or, better, sleep.' Another mother describes a more complex loss of interest:

> I had an episiotomy with my first child, and that caused quite a lot of pain after the birth. But the psychological effect was much greater, especially of breastfeeding. My body was no longer sexual. It was a functional thing for feeding a baby. It wasn't that the sexual sensations weren't there – although they were less – but my needs were so tied up with the baby and I suppose my needs were partly met by the baby. My breasts were not sexual. They were for the baby.
>
> **Janet, sons 8 yrs and 4 yrs**

There are many reasons why a breastfeeding woman may be less interested (or even completely uninterested) in sex. Breastfeeding completely changes her hormonal make-up, although nobody understands exactly what effect this has because it is so hard to separate out the hormone-induced changes from all the other variables.

Breastfed babies tend to feed more often than bottle-fed babies, and less predictably. Demand feeding is now considered the best way to feed, particularly in the early days when you are establishing the milk supply. Breastfed babies tend to need more night feeds or to continue night-feeding longer than bottle-fed babies. Some women find they can feed lying down, which makes night-wakings slightly less stressful.

Breastfeeding uses your energy to make as well as deliver the milk, and it cannot be shared. Overall, breastfeeding mothers are quite likely to be more tired than those using bottles, even though bottles can be more of a hassle.

Breastfeeding may satisfy some, or even most, of the mother's need for physical affection, and/or may leave her feeling 'touched out' – that she has had enough holding, pawing and pulling for one day. This does not mean she doesn't want a reassuring cuddle with her partner, but she may not feel up to the more protracted and intimate contact of making love. Many women say that during the period they were breastfeeding they simply could not bear to have their breasts touched by anyone other than the baby. Corinne found exactly this after the birth of her third child.

> It's very difficult to have a lot of sexual contact without it affecting your breasts. Sometimes you just don't want anyone else at you. You just feel mauled. Sometimes I even got part-way into love-making and said stop – and that was often why.
> **Corinne, daughter 10 yrs, sons 5 yrs and 7 m**

Breastfeeders tend to have less time away from the baby, either alone or with their partners. Unless you learn to express breast-milk (which can be very useful) or you (and the baby) are happy with an occasional bottle of formula, it can be very difficult to get an adult evening out.

Do try and get some designated time to yourselves as adults occasionally – if only within the house. And even if you cannot get out alone, do go and do adult things with the baby. A breast-feeding baby who still fits in a carrycot is usually very portable. Adult parties, meals with friends, restaurants, exhibitions, places of interest, parks or beaches are all possible if you are prepared to feed in public, though do be sensitive to local culture if you are abroad. Wear a baggy sweater or T-shirt and there is no reason why you should not feed anywhere, weather permitting. It can make a big difference to your state of mind to get out in the adult world.

Once breastfeeding is no longer your child's only form of food, you may be able to get out together during the day and get back for the evening feed (which is usually the last to go). You can even go to the cinema or theatre in the afternoon – though if you go out through what would normally be a breastfeed you may need to take extra pads or express a bit of milk, as the breasts fill up.

Breastfeeding usually creates or maintains a strong bond between mother and baby, which is in a sense an extension of the relationship in the womb. Weaning a baby through force of circumstance can be very hard for both baby and mother (and sometimes father, if he is brought in to do it). When it comes to a natural end – when the baby and mother feel ready – it may be a combination of slight sadness and relief.

> I really enjoyed breastfeeding and would not have done it any other way. But during the ninth month I slowly realized I had had enough – and I felt my son had too. He didn't really seem to mind being weaned. Shortly after he had stopped feeding, I realized I felt completely different. I had energy, I could run, I felt much more like the old me. It was as if the birth was finally over.
>
> **Jennifer, son 2 yrs**

This feeling that the birth is only fully completed with weaning makes some physiological sense, though it is not something all women feel. The mother's body is largely ruled by the baby's needs from conception until the end of breastfeeding. Menstrual periods will now return, if they have not already, and reduced sexual drive may slowly rise if the loss of libido is not due to other things like perineal pain or continued exhaustion.

It should now be easier to leave the baby with a good babysitter and get a few evenings out. If you have not been away from the baby so far this can be a bit daunting, but you may find that the minute you are out of the house you feel fine. Getting out and about as a couple again can make a world of difference to your relationship at home.

Effects on the Father

Some fathers love the sight of their partners breastfeeding, are delighted that their child is getting the best, and are generally happy with the whole business.

> I was very strongly in favour of breastfeeding and I did a lot –
> I hope I did a lot – to support it. On one occasion I had a
> fairly unpleasant argument with a man in a restaurant who
> tried to stop my wife breastfeeding. I didn't feel excluded. It
> made me feel very protective and paternal.
>
> **Mark, son 2 yrs**

Even if they are keen for the baby to be breastfed, however, some
fathers find the reality less easy. A few find it sexually off-putting
to have the baby at their partner's breast, but the most common
problem is jealousy.

Breastfeeding continues the special relationship between
mother and baby and the father may feel left out and jealous (of
either or both of them). At the same time he may feel displaced
from his partner's breasts, which can be particularly frustrating for
a man who is attracted by his partner's now larger breasts. He may
feel displaced from her body in general, and need to be reassured
that this phase is temporary and does not mean he is unloved.

> I was very elated by the birth. That didn't change my view of
> Sarah's body at all. It was when Kirsty [the baby] was very
> much attached to Sarah physically and emotionally that I
> found it more difficult. Suddenly Sarah's body was for the
> baby. I felt excluded. I didn't really expect that. You expect a
> more bipartisan arrangement. There's a baby that has access,
> but I expected an addition rather than a replacement. It
> sometimes felt as if the baby had access and I didn't. Once
> Kirsty was weaned, it began to change, but very gradually.
>
> **Malcolm, daughter 1 yr**

Meanwhile, incidentally, Malcom's partner Sarah was feeling
resentful at the fact that she had to get up round the clock to feed
the baby, while he did not!

The male inability to breastfeed makes some men feel inadequate in relation to the baby. It is certainly true that if a fully
breastfed baby is crying with hunger only its mother will do. And

sometimes even if it is not milk that is required, the breast may be the comfort the baby wants. But there are times when a baby is crying, perhaps for an unknown reason (like the dreaded 'colic'), when the father may be a better person to calm him. The smell of milk on the mother is not always helpful and after some time with an inconsolable baby she may herself start to get into a state, which sets up a vicious circle with the baby.

The more the father has been involved in learning about and establishing breastfeeding and the more he is involved with the baby, the less likely it is that there will be a disruptive level of jealousy. There is no point in the father competing with the mother, or vice versa. He has different things to offer: new ideas for playing, walks, a fresh shoulder, a different face above the changing mat, and so on. Even if it doesn't feel like it on some long breastfeeding evenings, babies need a lot other than the breast, especially as they get older. A mother may also want to try and give the father a bit of time alone with the baby – which also gives her a break.

Jealousy is sometimes subconscious and can lead men to behave in ways that are unhelpful, unsupportive or designed to draw attention back to themselves. Needless to say, this only makes things worse. So if either of you suspects that there is a problem with jealousy, try to talk about it (without accusing anybody). Open discussion and reassurance on both sides can stop the feelings festering and the ill-effects growing.

If this is your first child, breastfeeds can also be a good time to sit down together (though not perhaps for discussions about jealousy) and relax, chat, read or watch television. Your child's mealtimes will not always be this peaceful!

Effects on Love-making

We have already said that breastfeeding can affect libido – certainly in the woman and occasionally in the man. Parents often talk of sexual/psychological 'confusion' caused by breastfeeding. Are her breasts part of the sexual body or are they only for the baby?

Part of this problem is the way couples identify themselves as parents OR lovers rather than both (*see Parents 'Don't', page 139*). In fact, of course, the body is both sexual *and* reproductive and can carry the two roles simultaneously, within the confines of what is comfortable.

If your partner's breasts are uncomfortable or very full, or she just doesn't want them touched, you may need to adjust your position during sex to avoid them. Positions used in later pregnancy may be useful to keep pressure off the breasts.

The hormone oxytocin – which is involved in both sex and birth – is also involved in breastfeeding. It controls the milk let-down reflex, so breast stimulation, sexual arousal and sometimes orgasm can cause milk to leak (or occasionally spurt) from the breasts.

> Sex just seemed to be milk everywhere. Physically it was messy and psychologically it was too complicated for me. What was all this milk doing? He wasn't trying to suckle but he was getting some. It didn't seem to bother him at all. He just thought it was all quite understandable. He took it in his stride.
>
> **Susanne, daughter 2 yrs**

Some people do find the milk off-putting. As in Susanne's case, this can be as much because it is a reminder of the 'other' use for the breasts as because it is a bit messy. Milk leakage can theoretically be avoided by feeding the baby just before love-making, but you probably have enough trouble finding good times to make love without adding this to your list of conditions.

If you are not too bothered by a bit of milk (which incidentally does not sour and smell like cow's milk) it is probably easier just to accept this as part of post-childbirth love-making and keep tissues or a towel to hand.

Some men want to taste the milk (as do many women). If this is a matter of simple curiosity it should not cause any problems – and men may anyway get milk during foreplay if you are involving the breasts in sex. If the man actually wants to suckle, however, he should be warned that for some women this is one step too far in the confusion of the sexual and the maternal.

The way you both feel about her breasts may change as breast-feeding becomes more established and it is longer since the birth. What is off-limits at six weeks may be fine at six months. And when you stop breastfeeding, things may not instantly return to the way they were before you were pregnant. Breasts can become or remain more or less sensitive long after you stop feeding. So do keep talking and let each other know if your feelings change.

Parents 'Don't'

'The role of mother and the role of lover in our society seem to be totally opposed,' said one mother. Much less often, the same applies to fathers. The basic problem is the idea that parents – and especially mothers – 'don't'. This is ridiculous, of course, but it is well ingrained into many a subconscious.

For a man there may be a subconscious reluctance to make love to a mother; the connection being made with his own mother. Tim Kahn of Parent Link runs groups for fathers. He says,

> For some men there is a real confusion between their partners and their mothers, especially when their partners become mothers. Some men identify, sometimes relate to, their part-ners as if they were their mothers. It doesn't seem to happen so much in reverse, perhaps because the father is less closely identified with the child.

For a woman it is less likely to be any connection with her father that causes problems, than the more abstract idea that there is something wrong with mothers being sexual. Culturally, mother-hood is at the opposite end of the spectrum from the 'loose woman'; the ideal of motherhood being that presented by the vir-gin mother of Christ.

Men may also have a problem with role models. How many male heroes can you think of who were fathers? Most of them probably were, but the fact is considered irrelevant. Fathers of the previous generation do not generally fill the gap. Today's fathers probably want to be or are expected to be more involved than their own fathers were; their fathers were probably little involved with the children, and if they talked about sex with their sons at all, it would rarely have been about sex and parenthood. The sad fact is that our society is not very good at seeing sex as an integral part of family life.

The rise and rise of the child abuse issue may not have helped, either. Parents are made more self-conscious and even less comfortable with the idea of sex in the family, even though it is clearly between the two adults only.

Try to retain an image of each other as individual adults as well as parents. Calling each other 'Mummy' and 'Daddy' to the children makes obvious sense, but some couples fall into the trap of continuing this in private, often adding to the parent/partner confusion.

Whichever parent is at home the most may find it particularly difficult to switch roles from parent to lover. Many full-time mothers find it hard to click out of children and parent mode and into adult and lover mode. This is partly the old image problem – 'How can I feel sexy (or he find me sexy) with ketchup all over my shirt and puked-up milk on my shoulder?' – and partly having been part of a children's, rather than an adult's, world all day. It is exacerbated, of course, by the fact that there is always the possibility of having to switch back into parental role if a child wakes or needs something.

Parents are meant to be responsible and, according to Denise Knowles, a counsellor with Relate, sex does not always fit into our image of responsibility. Making love to make babies may be OK, but what about recreational sex? If you find yourselves taking everything too seriously, Denise Knowles says, take note: 'You may need to put the fun back into it.'

There is, of course, absolutely nothing wrong with parents having sex, and having it in any way they want to. A happy relationship between the parents (which will usually involve making love) is of benefit to the children as well. And the more relaxed you are with your own sexuality the more chance you have of bringing your children up to be happy with theirs. After all, where do people get the idea that parents 'don't', if not from their own parents?

Though you clearly do not want to flaunt adult sexuality in front of your children, children do need to see their parents being affectionate.

It may take a bit of getting used to, but sex IS a part of family life. Your sexuality and your parental role can co-exist.

> For the first two years of my son's life I found it hard to be sexy if I had any thoughts of him or the [parenting] day. Then one night we did something we had not done in years and made love on the stairs. Our son's door was just at the top of the stairs, and for a moment I felt awkward, even though I knew he was sound asleep. Then I thought – this is silly. Sex is a family thing. Without sex there is no family. Why should I feel awkward? And I haven't since.
>
> Natasha, son 3 yrs

Parents DO!

Where Should the Baby Sleep?

In the course of pregnancy and early parenthood you will probably hear or read strong views on where babies should sleep. The two extremes are: 'Cots are cages. The best and safest place for a baby is in bed with its mother/parents' and 'Family beds are unsafe and unhealthy. Babies should never be allowed to sleep in your bed.'

Ignore them both, and do whatever works for you and your baby. Some babies do not sleep well with two other bodies moving around them. Others like to snuggle up. Some find security in knowing this is where their parents sleep, others prefer their own cosy space to the large expanse of a double bed.

Adults vary, too. You may find it comforting to know the baby is right there; to be able to hear or feel her breathe without moving. On the other hand you may find you are being wakened by every sniffle or wriggle and getting no useful sleep at all. Some parents also worry about rolling on to the baby or the covers going over her head. You may need to watch your duvets and the baby's temperature, but unless you are drunk or drugged, you are most unlikely to squash her. Worrying about it may not, however, make for a good night's sleep.

Occasionally, parents clash over where the baby sleeps. Some fathers, in particular, dislike the idea of the baby in the 'marital' bed. In the early months it would seem sensible (even in sexual terms) to do whatever leaves you least tired. And in the event of a deadlock, perhaps whoever is doing most of the nighttime parenting should get the casting vote.

It is true that if your child sleeps exclusively in your bed well into toddlerhood, you might have trouble getting him out (though not necessarily). This is unlikely to be a problem with a tiny baby, and if a child comes into the bed occasionally it should not take too much to wean him off it.

Some couples do find a baby in the bed – or even in the room – a barrier to love-making. There is nothing wrong with making love with a small baby asleep in the room. An older child might be more off-putting. If he did wake up he might be concerned about what his parents were doing to each other, especially if they were making strange noises. You might find yourselves having to offer comforting explanations for which you were not fully prepared.

There are other rooms in the house where you can make love, of course, which can be a good idea occasionally – and may also make it quite clear to you how much of an inhibitor the child is, or is not. You might also want to agree that the baby should go into her own bed or bedroom at some specified age or stage. For example when she starts to sleep through the night, or a few weeks after weaning.

If you want your young baby close to you, but do not want her actually in your bed, you can of course put her in a Moses basket or carrycot right up next to your bed. This is a good compromise for some families – allowing easy access for checking and feeding, without worries or wriggles interfering with anyone's sleep.

Work

The division of domestic and money-earning work can be a real source of tension in your relationship after a baby is born. If you are under a lot of financial pressure the problems will be obvious. A new mother forced back to work by circumstance can be very unhappy indeed, and a father left suddenly as sole breadwinner may feel under enormous pressure and trapped in a particular job or occupation. But even where money is not the main issue, the arrival of a baby can throw the work/home balance into turmoil. In general, the more change the baby brings, the harder it is likely to be.

If one of you has always had the main career or been the primary breadwinner, while the other was more interested in the domestic front, then you may slip quite easily into sole career/breadwinner and at-home carer/partner. Equally, if you are both ambitious career people who get a full-time live-in nanny soon after the birth and continue your careers, this may cause relatively little tension – although you may not see much of your children or each other, and may both have to compromise eventually. The greatest, and most immediate, threat to the relationship tends to come when one partner feels forced into a particular role by the other (you should work/you shouldn't work/the mother of my children should be at home/I didn't marry a boring housewife, etc.). Or where one of you gives up a career you cared about while the other continues much as before, something that is increasingly common as more and more women have successful careers before motherhood.

Losing your job or career can be a real loss – even if it is done by choice. You may be quite clear that you are doing the right thing, and over the moon with your new baby. But you may still need to mourn the loss of your previous self – and all that went with it (*see Postnatal Depression, page 150.*)

Angela Martin, Relate counsellor and sex therapist, says today's new parents have grown up with the expectation of having it all. If they then give up a career to look after children, the reality is a shock: 'loss of role, of contact with the outside world, of having been seen as your own person. Loss of respect, perhaps loss of your own money and loss of time to yourself.'

The partner who becomes sole money-earner also has stresses to face. He (or she) has taken on a new financial responsibility and may feel trapped in a given job or career. On the whole, however, his or her role in society has been added to by becoming a parent, while the partner who gives up a career to be at home, though she or he has gained, has also lost.

Society's attitude to parents-at-home doesn't help. Suzanne (formerly a successful publisher) took her triplets, aged nearly two, on a routine visit to a speech therapist. The therapist asked how much both parents spoke to the children individually. Suzanne replied that during the week she was mostly alone with them, her husband coming in only after the triplets were in bed, and at weekends he was quite tired. She added that she was pretty tired too! The speech therapist looked at her with a completely straight face and said, 'But you're not working.'

This sort of reaction is not reserved for full-time or female parents-at-home. Ray job-shares, spending half the week looking after his two children:

> When I say at work that I am at home tomorrow, male friends say, 'Oh, feet up tomorrow then.' I have to put them right. Home is constant demands – 'I'm hungry, I need a pee, wipe my bottom,' ALL day. A lot of men don't appreciate what it is like. They may have stressful jobs but they don't recognize the stress levels of being at home with little children all day every day.

The sad fact is that careers and outside jobs are understood and respected. Childcare is not. This attitude has unfortunately become increasingly common as 1970s feminism and 1980s materialism have conspired to undervalue the home. Marsha usually works full-time, but took several months' leave after each of her two births.

> You get absolutely no respect when you are at home. YOU may know the house is still standing and the kids are developing, but there is no recognition. When I was on maternity leave, I had to go into the office for one day. I did something and a colleague said, 'thank you.' I was really surprised. You work very hard at home, but you get no feedback, no thanks.
>
> **Marsha, daughter 4 yrs, twins 2yrs**

All this does nothing for the parent-at-home's self-confidence or self-respect. Just as our physical self-image affects our relationship and sexuality, so does our social self-image.

The problem is at its most acute if these attitudes are shown by the 'working' partner, or if he or she is unsympathetic. Feeling valued is a vital part of a happy relationship, and a feeling of being misused can easily filter from the kitchen and sitting room to the bedroom.

Besides the loss of professional identity that can strike the parent-at-home, there is the reality of day-to-day caring for young children. The fact is that, however much you love your little one(s) and however satisfying caring for them may generally be, it is also extremely hard work, very stressful, and can be mind-blowingly boring. Reading the same board book for the twentieth time or wiping yet another baby meal from the floor is hardly anyone's idea of a stimulating experience – let alone one to make you feel sexy.

A male partner who works outside the home is especially likely to fail to understand the stresses of being at home. When the father becomes the full-time carer, the mother has usually spent at least a few weeks or months at home (though she may forget what it is like). Many fathers have never looked after their children alone for so much as a couple of hours, let alone days or weeks on end.

Peter McDonald wrote for *She* magazine under the headline, 'Men Haven't a Clue About Motherhood', describing the time when he had to take over his three children, aged 6 years, 21 months and 4 months, for three weeks when his wife went into hospital:

> I used to think I could cope with most things. My life as a surgeon has been one of constant activity and I have been accustomed to performing several tasks at once, such as stopping the bleeding, talking to a relative and thinking about my latest research project all at the same time.
>
> Until it happened, I always thought I was competent, a coper. But my self-assessment must have been wrong...
>
> In a rather smug middle-class way I have always prided myself on being a 'doer' at home – the sort of Home Counties Dishwasher and Occasional Nappy Man you meet in

Sainsbury's on Saturdays. So much part of our happy domestic scene did I consider myself that I would get irritated when my wife tried to fit me into her well-practised routines. So, when the call came, it was not as if I had never had an introduction course. That would have been some excuse for the chaos that followed...

Suffice it to say that by 10 o'clock at night...I fell unconscious into my bed. Never had I felt so tired. Not when I climbed the Himalayas and certainly not after a weekend of continuous hospital work.

When I visited my wife, who herself was suffering and looking awful, I would say, 'Darling, you look great considering!' In reply, without appreciating the asymmetry of our respective remarks, she would say, 'God, you look like death warmed up!'...

Now...As I climb on the Metropolitan line each morning at 7 a.m., giving the impression of a harassed commuter, I know who is the lucky one.

Another father, who often spends days at a time working away from home, was left alone with his one-year-old twins for 24 hours. At crack of dawn the following morning he was pleading with his wife to return because he 'hadn't had time to eat'.

The upshot is that a 'working' parent with a partner at home who gets back expecting a clean and tidy house, dinner cooked and on the table, a sleeping, sweet-smelling baby and a relaxed, interesting and sexy partner has another think coming. If he (or she) also expects to be able to come and go as freely as before, working late or going out for drinks, he or she is more than likely to return to a partner who is not only exhausted, stressed and covered in baby food, but resentful and stroppy as well – and not without reason.

Ruth Grigg of the Family Planning Association says that, after their first child was born, 'My husband and I made a rule – NO staying behind at work, NO late meetings, NO after-work socializing. It has worked so far. Men (or whoever is out at work) have got to understand that while they are out – you are working. Every extra minute they are not there is overtime for you.'

Clearly there will be times when some jobs require late working. This is not as often as many people like to think, but when it does happen the key is forewarning. The most crucial thing for a working partner to remember is to stick to what he or she says. If you have said you will be back at six, be back at six. If your child is old enough, he will be expecting you, and your partner may be relying on your return.

> If you have had a stressful day with the child, you focus on when you will have someone to help, someone to talk to. You have got your eye on the clock thinking – 'I've only got to survive the next hour, half-hour, 10 minutes.' If that person then fails to show up, if he is half an hour, even 10 minutes late, you're building up such a head of steam. If he then comes in and casually flops down without even apologizing for being late, you are ready to murder him. You may even have been waiting for him just to be able to go to the loo on your own.
>
> **Chrissie, son 2 yrs**

Over the first year or so of parenthood, most couples sort out their routines, expectations and children's bedtimes. This lessens the pressure on both partners – at least until you have another one. But occasionally, things do not settle down. Sometimes one or the other partner – more often the woman – finds she is not cut out for the role she has been given or given herself, whatever this may be.

It can be very hard to admit that your role is making you seriously unhappy – especially if that role is the one expected of your sex. For a man to say he can't take the financial responsibility and can't bear not seeing his baby all day is considered 'unmanly'; for a woman to say she is getting more and more depressed alone at home with her child carries fear of the 'bad mother' label. Women are sometimes caught the other way, too. In certain circles to give up a career to be at home full-time is to 'wimp out', becoming a useless, dependent woman.

Hard as it can be, you need to ignore all this nonsense and do whatever is right for you and your family. And try not to get caught in the guilt trap which is set for all parents – especially mothers. Penny Mansfield of the marriage and partnership research organization One Plus One says, 'Have the confidence to understand yourself, and say "This is the best parent I can be."' Unhappiness does not make for good parenting.

Penny herself took seven months after her first child was born to sort out her career/motherhood mix:

> I was very anxious to prove that she [the baby] wouldn't make any difference [to my career]. When she was seven months I remember thinking, no – it's gone. It will never be the same again. I am a mother that works, not a working mother. I felt incredibly relieved – and regretful that I hadn't realized earlier. Who was I trying to prove it to? Myself, I suppose.

Penny set about reducing her work-load and making her life more flexible so that she was more available for her child.

Judith, a barrister, had always intended to return to work when her baby was six months old. As the time approached and she began to look for childcare, she started to get unidentifiable pains and couldn't sleep. When her husband finally suggested she might prefer to stay home with the baby, the pains disappeared and sleep returned.

Other women need to go the other way.

> It took me two years to realize I had to get out of the house and restore some professional identity. I couldn't do it until I realized that my son was suffering because of the state I was in. My relationship with my partner had been suffering for some time. I resented the fact that he still had a career and came and went as an individual adult. I felt I had given up what was quite a successful and exciting career to become a mother and wasn't doing that very well. In the end, I found an excellent nanny share and went out to work part-time. We are all much happier.
>
> **Natasha, son 3 yrs**

I went back to work part-time when my daughter was six

months old. I think it made all the difference. Sex returned to normal. I had more time on my own, I felt normal, part of the human race again. I loved my baby but I couldn't bear being at home – especially in winter – with a baby who did nothing. I used to fight with my husband. I had to ask him for money which I had never done before. It was horrible. Even the baby seems happier now.

Sarita, daughter 1 yr

For men the problem most often comes later. Penny Mansfield again:

Men often find children of four or five more rewarding and by then they cannot avoid the child's disappointment. The child says directly, 'Daddy, why aren't you coming to my carol service?' which has much more effect than the mother saying, 'She'll be disappointed if you don't come to the playgroup open day.' Mothers who have not so far compromised their careers may also come up against this disappointment in the child and face the same problems as men.

The conflict can then arise between a job that is probably the basis of the family's finance (and perhaps the father's identity), and the desire for more time and flexibility. You may find you can squeeze much more of both without seriously affecting your career. It is amazing how work expands to fill the time available and how the macho work ethic makes people work far later and more rigidly than is absolutely necessary. And there may be others delighted to take over the 'task' of business trips abroad.

If you decide you need more drastic change, you may have to think about changing the kind of work you do, renegotiating your contract (could you job-share?) or simply taking what you need and being prepared for the possibility of others passing you on the career ladder – though this won't necessarily happen.

Some men find a decision not to compete, to get out of the rat race, hard to combine with their masculinity. It can lead to the same sort of loss of confidence and ill-effect on relationships that women suffer when they let ambition go. The issue is the same –

a matter of priorities and compromise, of working out what kind of balance will really work best for you and your family.

Neither partner should ever assume that work patterns CANNOT be changed because of employers or domestic finances. As far as employers are concerned, if you don't ask, you won't get – and some companies do have family-friendly schemes that men seem not to even know about, let alone take up.

At home, if one or both of you is really unhappy then everything has to be up for discussion. There is obviously a limit to how much money a family can give up in order to have one or other parent around more, but you may decide that some loss of income is the lesser of two evils. At the end of the day children need two reasonably relaxed parents more than they need new train sets.

Having said that, changing work arrangements is, of course, easier said than done, and almost always takes time. In terms of your relationship, just recognizing the problem can help. At least then you understand each other's feelings. And there may be little things you can do to help make up for work arrangements that are less than ideal – give the at-home parent half a day or an evening away from the kids, or the out-at-work-too-much parent a half-day alone with them. Meanwhile, if you can keep a really open mind about your job, you may eventually find a compromise that works.

Postnatal Depression

The baby blues, which often come around day four and last for a matter of days, are normal. They are nothing to worry about, requiring only understanding (*see page* 76). But if the depression gets worse rather than better and does not lift in a matter of a few weeks, it may be 'postnatal depression' (PND).

Postnatal depression is not well defined. It can be anything from a severe and longer-lasting version of the baby blues to a psychiatric disorder worthy of hospitalization. Between 10 and 20 per cent of women are thought to suffer from some form of PND, though many are never diagnosed. Not surprisingly, relationship problems and other social stresses make PND more likely.

Symptoms can be many and varied. They may include despondency and lethargy, a feeling of being unable to cope with the baby, anxiety, panic attacks (especially when trying to shop or travel on public transport) which can lead to fear of leaving the house, irrational fears, fear of harming the baby, unexplained aches and pains, sadness and frequent (often unexplained) crying, or constant irritability and tension, inability to concentrate or face even the simplest task, difficulty in sleeping or relaxing, poor appetite, and loss of interest in sex (though women can lose interest in sex after birth without this being caused by depression). Women also often feel guilty about the fact that they are not coping with motherhood, which only makes matters worse.

The cause of PND is unknown, though it is probably a mixture of hormonal and emotional factors. There is no instant cure, but if you/your partner is very low after the birth, it is important to recognize what is happening and seek help.

A woman who is depressed after childbirth (whatever you want to call it) needs a lot of practical and emotional help. She needs plenty of rest (even if she cannot sleep), to eat well (depressed women sometimes forget to eat), to be encouraged about her ability as a mother and her value as a person, NOT to be told to pull herself together. She needs no added stress (like moving house or making major decisions), to get out and see friends (though she may need a lot of support to do this), to be reminded that postnatal depression comes to an end and, perhaps above all, to be able to talk freely about her worries and feelings to an understanding and sympathetic listener – ideally perhaps a combination of her partner, another mother who has suffered postnatal depression, and an experienced counsellor (see Further Information for contacts). Ideally also, counselling or any doctor's appointments should involve her partner as well as herself.

Postnatal depression is often treated with anti-depressive drugs, which are intended to lift some of the symptoms, leaving you more able to recover from the causes of the depression. These will be prescribed by a doctor, and are best used in combination with talk or counselling. The tricyclic anti-depressants are given to women who are breastfeeding. The MAIOs should not be. A vitamin B_6 supplement or a multivitamin including B_6 may also help, though do not take more than 50 mg a day of B$_6$, as higher doses can affect the milk supply.

Living with someone who has postnatal depression may not be easy. Living without her may be even harder. A recent study found that over 50 per cent of the partners of women who had been admitted to a hospital mother-and-baby unit with severe PND were themselves clinically depressed. This highlights the fact that PND should be treated as a family problem. Fathers should be included in counselling and should seek support for themselves as well as their partners from the PND self-help groups (*see Further Information*).

Some new fathers get quite low after childbirth, regardless of whether their partners have PND. This has only just been noticed and is even less well understood than women's PND. Simon Lovestone, author of the research on PND partners, says, 'The problem is clearly greater in women, but I do think some men get postnatal depression.'

There is clearly not the physical element in men that there may be in women, but otherwise the reasons are perhaps similar – disruption of relationships, increased responsibility, loss of freedom, resurfacing of feelings about their own upbringing, emotional confusion when this 'joyous' time turns out to be difficult, and so on. New fathers may have fewer changes than new mothers. They also tend to have less support. Do seek out people to talk to (groups or individuals), and call the PND support groups if you need to (*See Further Information*).

Lack of sex can add to the problems surrounding PND. Loss of libido is a frequent symptom in PND mothers, and sexual interest may be one of the last things to return when she recovers. This can mean many months without sex.

I expected to have to wait a bit after the birth – perhaps two months. But even after three months Lorraine didn't want sex. We eventually tried and it hurt her. A few months more and it became obvious that things were not right. I came in one night to hear the baby screaming and my wife screaming back, she was having panic attacks in the supermarket and at church. Our son was already nine months old when PND was diagnosed.

Lorraine was put on anti-depressants and a psychiatric nurse came and gave us counselling for a year. Sex came back slowly. The nurse suggested starting with mild innocuous touching and fondling, then oral sex and mutual fondling, building up little by little. It seemed very sensible and it worked. I think it was about nine months after Lorraine was diagnosed that we had full sex.

I think Lorraine worried that I might not be satisfied. Maybe my sex drive isn't as high as some people's, but I just felt it was more important that Lorraine get better. You've got to be sensible. Now sex is as frequent and as good as before. There has been no permanent effect.

Mike, son 3 yrs

Sex is not always the last thing to return. Victoria Lehman, sex therapist and specialist in PND, says, 'I have had women say to me that if they give in and have intercourse, then the man will think they are much better and they will get less help and support.' Men may need to reassure their wives that they will not assume all is well just because she makes love with them.

The most crucial thing to remind yourselves throughout a period of PND is that it is never permanent. It WILL get better.

(More on surviving without sex and on restarting your sex life later.)

Communicating with Your Partner

In case you hadn't noticed, men and women are different, especially when it comes to sex. Physically this is obvious. But it is also true emotionally.

Jane Hawksley of Relate says, 'Men see sex as an affirmation, a confirmation that they are loved. Women see sex not as an affirmation or confirmation, but as something that happens when there is (already) love. Men and women come at sex from poles apart and can get their wires incredibly mixed.'

There are exceptions, of course, but generally men need sex to feel loved, while women need to feel loved in order to have sex. This is one of the keys to understanding each other, and it explains why a reduction in sex and lack of communication can lead so quickly to a dreadful emotional mess.

This is all generalization, of course, but take from it what applies to you...

Men who are feeling a lack of sex are feeling a lack of love. They need to be reassured that they are still loved, that lack of interest in sex is not lack of interest in them, that they have not been replaced by the baby and that the physical side of the relationship will return in time. They need to feel part of the new family, and have some attention paid to them. They also need physical affection, but they need to know roughly where they stand – is this foreplay or a platonic cuddle?

Women need to feel that their postnatal pain, exhaustion, loss of libido, etc. (whatever it is that is putting them off making love) is understood and appreciated. They need to feel loved and valued without feeling under pressure to have sex; they need to be able to give and accept affection without fearing that this will lead inexorably to more – or to the effort/guilt involved in having to rebuff their partner; they need time and attention paid to them as individuals. Peter Walker, who runs occasional postnatal fathers' groups, says men cannot not talk to their women and then expect to make love.

Talking is vital. Your lives may be running in parallel. Your days are probably more different now than they have ever been before. You need to know what the other one has been doing, and how he or she feels, otherwise you can get terribly out of touch.

Talking is also usually the only way to reassure, and to prevent or clear up misunderstandings. As we saw earlier, it is no good making assumptions about how the other one feels – you are very likely to get it wrong. And if you read the signs inaccurately too many times (e.g. a cuddle equals green light for sex/a cuddle equals pressure for sex), your partner may start to withdraw. Ask how he or she feels – and try not to jump down his or her throat when you don't like the reply. Keeping your cool can be very hard, especially if resentment has had time to build up before you talk.

You may need to be a bit formal about it – 'Let's talk about...You say how you feel and I won't interrupt. Then I'll say how I feel and you don't interrupt.' At least then you know your starting point.

Men are often less good at explaining their feelings than women, and less willing to reveal them to their partner or anybody else, as Janine discovered. She was feeling very low four months after the difficult birth of their baby; she could not face sex and resented her partner, who seemed unable to face the fact that things were not going smoothly.

> One day we went out with another couple who also have a young baby. I was talking to the other woman and the two men were talking. It turned out she was feeling very much the way I was – which made me feel a bit better.
>
> Her husband is like mine – all jolly and sociable and everything is fine. We – the two women – were talking quite openly and we got to saying, 'Oh sex – what's that? I remember that.' The men were horrified. They would have gone on pretending everything was just fine.
>
> **Janine, daughter 4 m**

The 'Ostrich Syndrome' is common, but not helpful. You need to be honest at least with yourselves and each other. And talking to other parents can be very helpful. You will almost certainly find others in much the same boat as you, and you may even be able to swap ideas on improving things.

Coping with Lack of Sex

It is extremely common for the postnatal weeks or months to be a sexual desert. Jerri Thoman, an antenatal teacher and breastfeeding counsellor, says we should keep it all in perspective, 'The childbearing and breastfeeding years are a very small part of your life. When you are in the middle of it, it doesn't feel like that, but it actually all happens very quickly. We need to take the long view.'

Putting pressure on for sex or allowing yourself to be pressured can be very counterproductive. Women need to learn to say no while making sure he realizes it is sex, not him, that is being rejected. Men need to realize that women are often not very good at saying no, and the result may be that she does it and hates it (and possibly hates you and herself as well), or she says no and feels guilty about it, neither of which is very helpful in the long run.

The first thing to do is to talk (*see Communicating With Your Partner, page 153*). If you can openly discuss the lack of sex – and perhaps even laugh about it – it will be a lot easier to cope with. If you can put yourselves on the same side in the situation rather than lined up against each other, it will make a huge difference both to your current happiness and to your chances of an easy return to love-making when the time is right.

Feeling you are 'in it together' can be easier if you are both very involved with the children. Susan and David, both of whom work from home, produced four children in five years. They both say sex was very scarce during this time, but that their relationship 'just kept blossoming'. Their interests were not divided by the arrival of children, but brought together.

> We are both very involved with the family. We spend almost all our time and energy on the family, and even when we are alone we talk mostly about the family. Our relationship has stayed very close and warm and intimate – and got more so.
>
> **David**

It is vital to maintain intimacy. Many relationships rely on sex for this intimacy and, when it is missing, there is a danger of losing the closeness as well. This is especially true if cuddles are assumed to be foreplay and are therefore avoided or rebuffed.

There needs to be a clear understanding that cuddles and kisses are not an invitation to, or pressure for, sex. They need to be taken and enjoyed for what they are (and they are very important). What happens next must be as optional as if the cuddle had not happened.

Massage can be a useful form of non-sexual physical contact. Take it in turns to give each other anything from a relaxing shoulder rub to a full-body massage, depending on how much time, energy and expertise you have. Once again, never assume this will lead to sex. (*See Further Information for books on massage, and Appendix B for non-sexual sensuality.*)

It may sound unromantic, but often the best way to find out if someone wants to make love is to ask: 'How do you feel about making love?/Might you feel up to making love?' Then at least she (or he) is given space for a reply. Which, if not yes, might go along the lines of, 'Sorry, I don't, but I would love a good cuddle/I do like having your arms around me.' It all sounds very stilted on the page, but the point is to give each other room to manoeuvre without rejection or guilt.

As far as physical sexual need is concerned, sex therapists often start by trying to make individuals take responsibility for their own, rather than each other's, sexuality. Therapist Jane Hawksley explains:

> I say to men – what did you do before you were married (or cohabiting)? My guess is you masturbated. You may need to do that again. Take care of that basic sexual need yourself for a while...
>
> I say to women – an erect penis is not your responsibility. It just means he desires you. It may not even mean he wants sex. Women often can't cope with an erect penis. Our culture brings women up to feel they have to do something about it...
>
> I say to men – if you ignore an erection, it will fade away. He has to come to terms with the idea that he can be aroused and does not have to do anything about it.

Some couples find the idea of masturbation (male or female) difficult to deal with. They may feel guilty about it. There is no need. There is nothing wrong with masturbating, and at times of sexual differences, separation, or sexual stress it can be useful.

Jane Hawksley says, 'For women, masturbation does not reduce your sexual drive and it won't do any harm. It may allow you to get in touch with your sexual feelings again, and has a guaranteed outcome. It can help build up your confidence again that you are still a sexual being.'

Men sometimes worry about the fantasies they may have while masturbating. Sex therapists say everybody fantasizes and it is perfectly healthy. It doesn't matter what your fantasies are (although if they are violent or unpleasant you may want to try and find a more benign one). Fantasies are only a problem if you start to want to turn them into reality.

Some couples, like Sam and Camilla, are able to come completely to terms with masturbation and fantasy within their relationship:

> When I feel I need to release fluid I need to do it, so I get on with it. I can do it in bed if I want to. I don't expect (or want) my wife to do anything about it. Or I would say to her, 'I need to be alone for a while,' and she would understand. It did take time to get to this. It was something that became acceptable in our relationship, not something that was there from the start. We talk a lot. It did help through pregnancy and after the children were born. We talk about our fantasies too. She knows mine and I know hers. There is nothing wrong with thoughts.
>
> After the children were born, I just used to say, 'Are you ready yet?' or 'Do you fancy...?' She started off by saying, 'No – I'm not ready yet,' or 'I'm a bit frightened,' so we just waited. The first time it was about four weeks, the second it was seven weeks. The second time, she actually said – 'I feel sexy now.' I'm sure it makes a difference that I am quite gentle and Camilla knows she can control it. If I go in too far, she knows she can say stop. Some men think strong thrusting is the only way to make love.
>
> We are unusual I suppose. We talk about it. Our friends talk about it. So there is just no real issue about it.
>
> **Sam, sons 3 yrs and 1 yr**

It is important to keep the channels for sexual contact open. If the channels for affection are there, these can be quite easily converted. But Penny Mansfield says no sex should not become a habit. It is worth bringing the subject up now and again.

Try not always to bring it up at midnight, and be careful not to withdraw affection or attention if your partner is still not ready. Be willing also to make an effort to ensure that if she (he) agrees to make love, she (he) enjoys it. This may require asking what your partner feels up to or wants.

Equally, do not be put off saying yes to sex with provisos: Yes, if you don't go in too far; Yes, but I'm exhausted, so you'll have to make a bit more of an effort/be patient if I am slow in getting going, etc. Do not dismiss non-penetrative sex. There is a great deal you can do without penetration (mutual masturbation, oral sex, anything you like).

It is quite possible for couples to survive without sex for many months – especially if there is a reason that is well understood by both of you – and if communication is not lost. Mark's son, Jake, was born with a serious congenital disease and was in and out of hospital throughout his first 15 months of life:

Sex stopped totally. It did not start again until two or three months after Jake's last operation, in other words, about 18 months after the birth. It also coincided with an end to breastfeeding (which had been prolonged because of his condition). It [no sex] was understandable. I felt frustrated – not angry, but perhaps wishing for something better, thinking, 'Oh Gosh, how much longer is this going to go on?' It did cause tension in the relationship but it is difficult to separate that from other tensions because everything was so pervaded by Jake's condition.

The lack of sex was a problem, but not an over-riding one. It never meant I wanted to throw the marriage away or anything. I masturbated perhaps a bit more than usual. And there was always the prospect of its return. I never doubted that our sex life would return. I kept pressing – no, not so much pressing as enquiring, trying it on, until Melissa felt up to it. It wasn't really surprising that that time came when Jake's condition was settling and we could be a bit more relaxed about him.

Once we did start again, we quickly got back into the way of enjoying sex, and it got very good. If anything it is better than before.

Now we're thinking about another baby.

Mark, son 2 yrs

Hanging on to the fact that your sex life WILL return can be very important. One of the biggest problems is when parents (especially fathers) think that this is how it is going to be from now on. It isn't. Sexuality WILL return. And if you can keep communication and intimacy going, it will return much more easily.

If you should get beyond a year after the birth and the end of breastfeeding, with no sex at all, no obvious reason for it, and no prospect of a return, this may be the time for a really serious talk and a concerted effort to change things. If you still find you are having a lot of difficulty, you may need some help. Sex therapist Jane Hawksley says, 'It's a bit like leaving a car in the garage for a year. You may not be able to just get in and drive it again. It may need servicing.'

Returning to Sex

See also …And Then There Were Three (earlier in this chapter) and The First Time (in Chapter 7).

'For your sex life, you really need a one-to-one relationship,' says David, the father of four children under five mentioned earlier.

We have four other people to consider. We have to remove the Duplo [bricks] from our bed before we can get in. We have no private space of our own. For the last few years that hasn't mattered – You don't have to have sex, and for us it has been almost irrelevant – But now that we have completed the family, we are actually thinking of having a room, perhaps with a four-poster bed – something a bit romantic – that is just ours. You get to the point where you have to do that sort of rather self-conscious thing...we have to reclaim our own space.

Different couples will, of course, have different ways of reclaiming their space and their sexual relationship. David's general relationship did not suffer as a result of the lack of sex, and communication lines were kept wide open. This makes any return much easier.

If you have had no sex at all for a year or more and your relationship has suffered; if affection has died with the sex life and you are not talking as well as you might, you may need help. You may, as it were, need to take the car to the garage for servicing.

Sex therapists usually suggest starting slowly. First – and throughout – you will need to talk. You will need to share your feelings – not only about sex, but about life in general. If you are not sharing day-to-day life you will find it a lot harder to share good sex.

One way to start the physical revitalization is to ban sex for a while. Decide that there will be no intercourse for a number of weeks, or – perhaps better – a number of sessions of time together. At the very beginning, you may want to ban all genital contact. The idea is to take the pressure off, and allow yourselves time and space to remember why you wanted to make love to each other in the first place.

You will need to set time aside for yourselves – quite specifically – so you can relax and take things slowly. You need to be able to separate yourselves from being parents and allow yourselves to be a couple again. You may have to be quite formal about giving yourselves time for 'sessions' to revitalize your sex life. It is the turn of your (sexual) relationship to be given some priority.

Start with kissing and cuddles. Perhaps do what you used to do before you first slept together (if you can remember what that was!). Sex therapists point out that kissing can be extremely intimate and loving and that, when there are difficulties in a relationship, kissing is often abandoned even while sex (of a sort) remains.

You may want to undress each other – something long-term couples often stop doing – or have a bath or shower together. Massage can be very good (even just shoulders or back) if you have used it before or are prepared to try. You need to rediscover each other's body, and get to know and accept it as it is now. You need to remember how to be physical with each other outside any old, established pattern of foreplay, or feeling of pressure for 'full' sex.

Move on to gently touching and caressing – perhaps initially excluding, and then including, the genitals. Sex therapists often suggest taking it in turns to touch each other, saying or showing the other one what works best. Even if you knew each other's preferences inside out before childbirth, it is quite possible that things have changed.

If you have never communicated very directly about sex, a session like this may feel very awkward at first. But you could both learn a lot. You might want to sit with the 'receiving' partner in front of the 'giving' one, both with your legs out so the 'receiver' can sit between the legs of 'giver' and lean against him/her. This allows you to be physically close without having to cope with eye contact while you overcome any initial embarrassment.

It is vital that the ban on sex remains in place at this stage. You may find this frustrating. If you are both starting to feel frustrated – good – then you will really want it when the ban is lifted!

This sort of touching may naturally move on to masturbating each other (perhaps one after the other rather than trying to do it at the same time), or perhaps oral sex or whatever you want and find acceptable. Non-penetrative sex is much ignored and underestimated and, especially if your problem has been one of perineal pain or fear of penetration, it can be very useful indeed.

Finding new ways of giving yourselves sexual pleasure can be very helpful. You may have been stuck in a sexual rut (to coin a phrase) even before the baby was born, and this hiatus in the relationship may help you get out of it. There are a number of sexual self-help books that might be useful. Some are specifically designed to help you 'rekindle the flame', or have sections on this. Some of them can seem a bit daunting at first, but if you take from them what you – both – want, and ignore the rest, you may find them very useful (see Further Information).

Making love in new ways DOES NOT have to mean anything particularly weird or wild. In fact, it may mean doing less, or taking it more gently (see Appendix B). It may mean being happy not always to have 'full' intercourse. You can take it in turns to do things for each other instead of always aiming for the (often elusive, or even illusory) simultaneous orgasm. If you do go for simultaneity and it doesn't happen, you could do something afterwards to bring the other one to climax if he/she wants it. The more satisfying sex is for both of you, the more likely you both are to want to do it.

There are various positions for full sex as well, of course (and various times and places). The traditional man-on-top 'missionary' position is often the least satisfactory for a woman – especially if she needs clitoral stimulation as well as penetration (as most women do) to reach orgasm.

The woman can go on top – either sitting or leaning forward on to her partner; the man can enter from behind her, leaving his hands free to reach her breasts or her clitoris; she can sit on his lap facing him; you can do it over the edge of the bed; or you can both lie down and find the various (more relaxed) ways to make it work. One example is for the woman to lie on her back with her knees up over his body, which lies at 60 or 90 degrees to her. If you are interested in different positions, have a look at Appendix B and experiment. Jettison ones that don't work for you, and enjoy the ones that do. Needless to say, there are books full of positions if you want to experiment more fully.

Some couples find sex toys (most commonly a vibrator), sexy clothes, films or magazines useful in rekindling sexual desire. There is nothing wrong with any of these, but ONLY if you are BOTH completely comfortable with them. One partner doing something that feels wrong for them will not help you redevelop a good sexual relationship.

If you are interested in trying something like this for the first time, ask your partner (gently) how he/she feels about it. You may be surprised. You can also leave the question open for the future, by saying that if he/she ever does get interested, to let you know. People's sexual interests and (dis)inhibitions do change (but don't pressurize!).

If you are going to try something very new, or something one of you is not quite sure about, be prepared to stop in the middle, and don't take it too seriously. A fit of giggles over a piece of lace or a vibrator may actually be rather good for your sex life.

Sex, after all, should not be taken too seriously.

If things have been bad enough that one or both of you has considered looking elsewhere for sexual (or emotional) satisfaction – or perhaps has even done it – you may have an extra barrier to overcome. If you are prepared to make an effort – and seek help if necessary – you may well find that you can fill the gaps in your life by improving life at home rather than gambling with the happiness of the whole family by 'playing away' from home.

You are most unlikely to recapture those first heady days of love and lust way back when you were first together. No normal human being could sustain this over a lifetime, let alone while continuing to function as a parent and an employee. You can, however, find something just as good, and much longer lasting. If you cross the desert and come out the other side, the chances are your relationship will be stronger and better.

10

DOING IT ALL AGAIN
SECOND BABIES AND BEYOND

Once you have recovered from the first round, or even if you haven't, statistics suggest you will probably start all over again. This time you will have a much clearer idea what to expect, although it is surprising how fast you forget.

You have already made the transition from partners to parents, from individuals to family. But you now have your first child to care for and consider. In some ways the second time round is easier; in others, more difficult. It is certainly going to be different.

No two pregnancies are the same and no two babies are the same. If you had a lot of problems the first time, they will not necessarily repeat themselves. If you have so far had an easy ride, you may be being lulled into a false sense of security.

Needless to say, much of what was said about pregnancy, birth and parenthood in the book so far applies equally to second and subsequent occasions, but the following will give you a few ideas about how things might differ.

Conceiving a Second Child

A child may seem like one of the best forms of contraception available, but parents do manage to conceive again. Trying to get pregnant may push love-making up your list of priorities and improve your sex life, especially if you normally find contraception a nuisance. For some, however, trying to get pregnant makes sex a chore. If you think one or both of you is feeling pressured to perform in order to conceive, do talk about it. Misunderstandings can easily arise and if you are not careful you can get into a vicious circle of assumptions, worry and unsuccessful sex. Even if you conceived immediately the first time, you will not necessarily do so this time, so try to relax and not panic if it takes a few months to happen.

Pregnancy

Second time round you are not on a constant journey of the unexpected, jumping for the pregnancy book or the phone at every twinge. But it may be very difficult to look after yourself well, to get time even to think about the new baby, to eat properly and especially to get enough sleep.

Non-pregnant partners, family and friends tend to be a lot less attentive during a second pregnancy. Women may have to remind their men that they are pregnant and need help and extra rest just like last time. Partners should try not to need reminding too often!

Much of what was said in the Tiredness section (*see Chapter* 8) applies here, too. The mother is growing a baby inside her as well as whatever else she is doing, so the father will need to increase his domestic load as well. And if Daddy is not already an acceptable alternative to Mummy for the older child, now is the moment to change this. In pregnancy, labour and the early postnatal period, Mummy is not always going to be available, and having two trusted parents may make it easier for the child to share them with the new baby.

If the last pregnancy was a sexual desert, that does not mean this one will be. But equally, if you were all over each other for nine months the first time, you may be in for an unsexy shock. Pregnancies can be poles apart, especially in sexual terms – and there are no rules about which way round this happens. Men's sexual reactions are likely to be less variable, unless there is a special difference, like whether each pregnancy was planned or not.

Second pregnancies may feel as though they are progressing more quickly. The body has been pregnant before and it seems to react faster to doing it again. You are likely to feel bigger and more pregnant earlier.

So long as nothing went terribly wrong the first time, you may now feel a bit more confident about the process of making a baby. If sex came to a standstill last time for fear of hurting the baby, the second pregnancy may be easier. If you had sex at all in your first pregnancy, you may also now have some ideas about what works for you in pregnant sex – though, do remember, it won't necessarily be the same.

You probably won't have either the time or inclination to read as much about pregnancy the second time round as you did the first, but do glance back and try to go to an antenatal refresher course. Medical policy and practice are changing very fast in maternity services, and it is also amazing how quickly and how much you forget. With luck, a class may also provide you with a new postnatal support group of parents with similar-aged children.

Birth

Statistically, the chances are that your second birth will be easier. Second labours are generally shorter and require less intervention. You have a greater chance of escaping an episiotomy or a tear, or at least of having much smaller ones than last time. Unless you had major problems first time round, medical staff are likely to be more relaxed during a second or third birth, and so you may have more freedom to do it your own way.

If your first birth was difficult, traumatic, or there was a medical emergency, you may be very worried about doing it again. Discuss this with each other and with your midwives or doctor. Ask if the kind of problems you had last time make it more likely that you will have difficulty this time, and tell them which aspects of the birth worry you most. If you had a Caesarean the first time, talk to the medical staff about why it was performed and what it means for this delivery. Many women do now have vaginal births after a Caesarean.

Even if the first birth was not especially difficult, there may be one thing you do not wish to repeat, or that still bothers you. This is worth discussing, both between you and with your professional carers. You could also put it in your birth plan. If your particular sensitivity is known, everyone is more likely to make a special effort to help you through it.

Because second births are generally faster than first ones, they can also be 'bumpier'. You need to remember that you may not have hours to set things up, organize older children, get to the hospital, discuss pain relief, etc. and that contractions may suddenly get tougher without the slow progression more characteristic of a first labour.

The speed of second labours makes it more likely that you will manage without major pain-relieving drugs. But it also means that if you definitely want an epidural you need to say so quite early on, or you may find you have passed the point where one can be inserted.

Second and third births are considered to be medically the safest and most predictable. This is, however, still labour and birth, and it is worth keeping an open mind about what it will actually be like on the night.

Parenthood

If you were tired last time...Many parents say two children is more than double the work and, at least at first, it can mean that both partners have their hands full of children and there is nobody left to do anything else.

Your second child may have a quite different character from your first, but you will probably still find caring for this one easier than you did when you were a total novice. Now, however, you also have your first child to think about. You may have two children waking in the night and your first child is likely to need a lot of support and reassurance in the weeks and months after the new baby arrives – just when you have least to give.

Get as much help as you can. And remember that even with two children, you will get the routines sorted out eventually. All the advice earlier in this book – about tiredness, sharing the load, talking, keeping up affection, etc. – all apply just as much, or even more, this time. You may not have so much of an identity crisis, but time, and perhaps money, will be at even more of a premium. Priorities may need rethinking again.

With any luck, returning to your sexual relationship should be easier – though this obviously depends on how the birth went and whether your sexual relationship reached a satisfactory plateau between babies. Although new problems are less likely after a second birth, they can happen and you may want to refer back to relevant sections of this book or check the Further Information chapter.

Do not expect the return to sex be quicker than the first time round, however. Sheer exhaustion and acute lack of time may ensure that it is not. Don't rush it. Hopefully, you will be sustained by the knowledge that you got through last time, and so you should be able to get through this time. Both or all your children will get older and easier and you will have more time and energy for your adult relationship again.

Summary of Part III

- Loss of interest in sex after childbirth, usually on the part of the mother, is very common. It can last many months but it is temporary.
- Loss of interest in sex is NOT loss of love. Rejection of sex is not rejection of the other person.
- Pressure, guilt and worry only make the situation worse.
- Sex is not obligatory.
- Masturbate if you need/want to. There is nothing wrong with it.
- It is quite normal to take anything up to a year to get your sexual relationship back to anything like 'normal'.
- The 'normal' you return to may not be the same as your pre-pregnancy norm.
- Quantity is often down, but quality may be up.
- It is vital to retain physical and emotional communication whether or not you are having sex: keep cuddling and be quite clear that cuddles do not mean an invitation to or pressure for sex.
- Talk to each other; openly, honestly, but kindly.
- The sexes are different. In general, men need sex to feel loved, women need to feel loved to have sex.
- Pain during intercourse in the months after childbirth is surprisingly common. It usually clears up by itself. If it does not, seek help – when you are ready.
- Breastfeeding can reduce vaginal lubrication and make you feel dry. Try KY Jelly and/or spit.
- The more your responsibilities and problems are shared and decisions taken together, the better your relationship and sex life are likely to be.
- Fathers who are involved with their children tend to make both themselves and their partners happier.
- Parents do have sex and (if they want to) should have sex. Sex is part of family life.
- The postnatal period may seem interminable but it is temporary. Babies change, adults sort themselves out and sex returns.
- Second or third time round is usually easier – though there is not necessarily more sex.

EPILOGUE

Suffice to say that, for all the difficulties they may bring, the vast majority of parents would not be without their children for anything – except perhaps for the odd couple of hours now and then!

POSSIBLE CAUSES OF PAIN DURING INTERCOURSE

'Superficial' Pain

(i.e. on the surface of the perineum or the vaginal wall)

Infection

If the wound is red, has pus in it or is smelly – or if you suspect an infection even though none of these signs is present – seek medical attention.

Narrowed Entrance to the Vagina (narrowed introitus)

If you are off sex generally and find it hard to get aroused, the feeling of tightness may be due to this and will be temporary. But if even complete relaxation and full arousal leaves the hole too small, you may have been stitched too tight.

If the narrowing is slight it is possible for it to stretch with use. Some women are advised to do this by having sex – hardly an option if sex is really painful (and beware of putting up with pain, it can lead to psychological sexual problems later). Sex therapists sometimes suggest using 'dilators' or 'trainers' – a set of penis-shaped objects ranging in size from a finger-width up. Not everyone is happy about using these, and you would need to take advice about whether they were suitable in your case. Your own fingers might be a more acceptable alternative. If all else fails, you may need to be restitched more loosely.

A *Lump, Loop or Layer*

Imperfect stitching can leave you with:

- A lump or ridge of scar tissue
- A skin bridge – a loop or a thin area of skin – usually at the back of the vagina where the lips (labia minora) meet. It may feel as though it could tear easily.
- A scar that pulls to one side – perhaps because a mediolateral episiotomy has been started in slightly the wrong place (i.e. not on the midline – *see Figure 1, page 20*).

Any of these can make the stretching and movement involved in sex uncomfortable.

Scar problems sometimes settle down with time (it may be months or occasionally years). They may be treated with specialist physiotherapy (usually ultrasound), or recut and resewn.

A *'Spot' of Pain*

If you can put your finger on an exact spot and say, 'This is where it hurts,' then there are a few possible problems:

- Neuromata (trapped nerve endings) – this is when a nerve is trapped in the scar and the ending is exposed. You – and anyone examining you – should be able to put a finger on an exquisitely tender spot. The pain should go if the pressure is moved even a millimetre or so either side. Once found this would normally be cut out, although some physiotherapists may try to desensitize it with ultrasound.
- Granulomata – these are little areas of scar that have not healed properly. It will be a sore, probably red, patch. It might heal up on its own in a year or so, but is more quickly solved by cauterization with silver nitrate to seal it. This often requires no anaesthetic, although a local may be used if necessary.
- Endometriotic spot – very rarely, a little bit of tissue from the lining of the womb (endometrial tissue) gets caught in the scar. This will be more tender during your periods (if you are having them again) and may look bluish under the skin. The 'spot' would normally be cut out.

Deep Dyspareunia

If you have pain at the top of the vagina or in the pelvis in general during intercourse, check for other symptoms. Discharge that smells unpleasant and fever would indicate a possible infection. If you think you might have an infection, do not delay seeing a doctor. This needs to be cleared up so that it does not spread.

Miscellaneous Superficial or Deep Dyspareunia

If none of the above matches your case, your problem may still be physical and a good doctor, midwife or physiotherapist may be able to find it. Otherwise, it is possible that the root cause is psychological. Your mind may have decided it cannot cope with sex at the moment and your body has found an effective way of stopping you from doing it.

A rule of thumb for separating physical and psychological pain is that if the pain is clearly identifiable and at a specific site, then it is probably physical. If it is more generalized it may be either physical or psychological.

Psychological causes are, of course, subconscious, and they create a pain that is perfectly real and not something the person can simply decide to stop feeling. If you think your problem is psychological – and the pain persists even once you have realized this – you need a good sex therapist.

The cause of the problem will be different for each person (and there may be several causes), but a few of the more common problems are listed below in case they give you a spark of recognition.

- Belief that the perineum is mutilated (usually causes superficial pain). Try looking in a mirror.
- Trauma from the birth – especially if you felt mistreated.
- Birth trauma rekindling past sexual trauma (e.g. rape, child abuse).

- Fear of getting pregnant again.
- Mothers 'don't' (the madonna syndrome).
- Problems in your adult relationship (father jealous of baby, etc.).

All these are looked at in more detail in Chapter 9.

ALTERNATIVE SEXUAL POSITIONS AND PRACTICES

Here are a few suggestions for positions and practices that might be useful during pregnancy and after childbirth. It may sound a bit clinical written down, but it may give you a few starting points if you need them. Adjust, ignore and invent to suit yourselves. In the end trial and error is the only way. If anything gets uncomfortable for either of you (physically or psychologically), do not suffer in silence. Talk it through and try something different.

You may want to have a few extra pillows, cushions or a beanbag handy. They might come in useful, especially in the latter part of pregnancy.

Intercourse

Variations on the Missionary Position/Man on Top

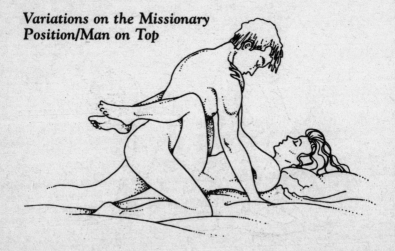

Man on top can be adjusted to take account of a bump, sore breasts or a Caesarean scar. He can simply take all his weight on his arms or he can keep his upper body more upright while her legs are held up in the air. Try some wriggling around and see what you come up with. The disadvantages of these positions are that the man's hands are generally not available for much other than supporting his own weight, pressure on the perineum is likely and the woman is on her back (which may not be the best position in later pregnancy or the early postnatal period).

Rear Entry

The man can kneel behind the woman, who can be on all fours. This avoids pressure on breasts and/or bump, gives easy access for the man (or woman) to the clitoris and/or breasts and puts less pressure on the perineum than the missionary position. This may be useful if the perineum is still a little sore after the birth. Rear entry allows deep penetration, however, so if you are trying to avoid this be careful. If the woman is pregnant, the man should be sure he is not putting his weight on her back.

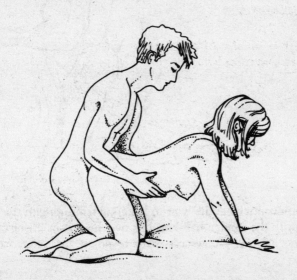

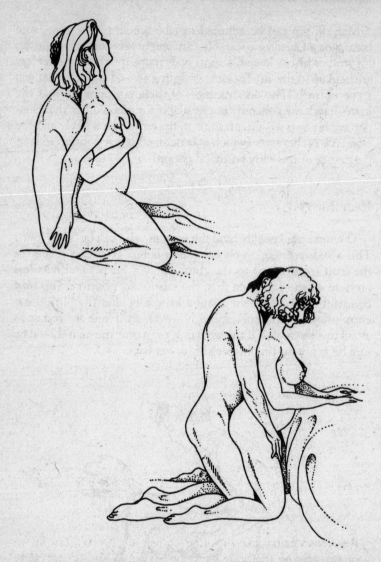

Variations include: the woman kneeling semi-upright; the man sitting with the woman half-kneeling over his legs or sitting on his lap. Kneeling on pillows can help to adjust for differences in height.

178

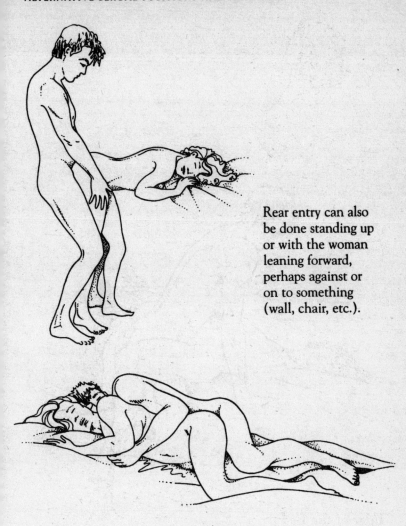

Rear entry can also be done standing up or with the woman leaning forward, perhaps against or on to something (wall, chair, etc.).

Rear entry lying down is often known as 'spoons'. You lie on your sides facing the same direction. You may end up not quite slotted together like spoons, as the man may want to move round a little to be able to get inside better and the woman may want to tip slightly on to her back or front and raise or part her legs in different ways.

179

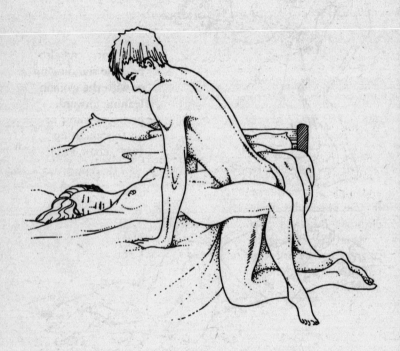

Edge of the Bed

The woman can sit on the edge of the bed or lie on her back with her legs over the edge. The man kneels on the floor so he is between her legs. She can vary how much she sits up or lies back according to the size of the bump or how she and her partner are most comfortable. This also keeps weight off breasts and bump.

Sides

You can both lie on your sides facing each other, then wriggle around until it works! A good one if you are tired. It can also be done from behind (*see Rear Entry, page 179*) in 'spoons' position.

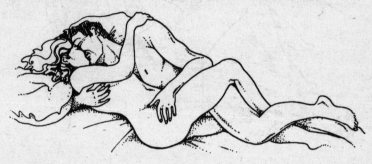

Woman on Top

The man lies on his back and the woman kneels astride him. This keeps all weight off her and allows her to control the depth and angle of penetration, etc. It gives reasonable access to the clitoris and breasts.

Variations include the man sitting partially or completely upright or the woman leaning over him to almost lie on top.

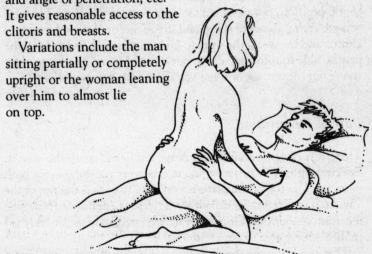

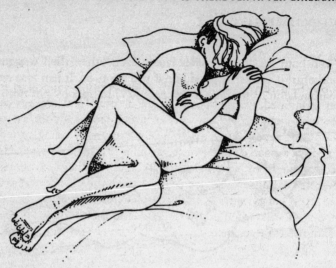

Lying Down

The woman can lie on her back or prop herself up slightly with her knees up. The man lies on his side and curls his lower half under the 'bridge' made by her legs so he can enter her. This is quite a gentle position, not designed for deep or hard thrusting. Useful if you are trying to avoid these and if you are tired. Good access to clitoris and breasts. If the woman is uncomfortable on her back she may be able to turn partially to one side. This can also be good for trying out tantric sex or some variation on it (*see page 184*).

Partial Penetration

There is no rule that says penetrative sex has to go all the way in. Penetrating just into the vagina can be very pleasurable for both partners. The top of the penis is very sensitive, as is the rim of the vagina. If you definitely do not want deeper penetration, however, a certain amount of self-control may be necessary as you may get quite a strong urge to penetrate further.

This can, of course, be done in any position, but the one immediately above or variations upon it are some of the easiest.

Non-penetrative Sex

Oral Sex

This can be a very good alternative to penetration when that is either prohibited, worried about or not desired. Oral sex can be done simultaneously (69) but you may find it more comfortable to do it one at a time. This is a useful, gentle way of bringing a tired or pregnant woman or one whose vagina is dry due to breastfeeding to orgasm, or of bringing a man to orgasm without involving the female genitalia. Some people do not like the taste of oral sex or are only happy with it under certain circumstances. Some women do not like their partners to come in their mouths. If you have not tried oral sex before, you might want to talk about it first.

Manual and Non-manual Stimulation

You can masturbate each other simultaneously or alternately. Or one of you may not want to receive this time. Extra lubrication such as spit or *KY Jelly* can be useful, since hands do not produce their own and it can all get rather dry (especially for breastfeeding women). Watch out for fingernails and try to agree to be open about what works and what doesn't.

Alternatively the man can put his penis high up between the woman's legs – keeping it between her legs rather than up into the vagina. If she has her legs together this creates the necessary pressure on the penis and can also give good clitoral stimulation to the woman. The man can also reach orgasm with his penis between his partner's breasts.

Tantric Sex

The Indian Tantric religion involves the search for ecstasy and has a large sexual element (the *Kama Sutra* is part of the Tantric tradition). This may not seem to have much direct relevance to 1990s Western love-making, but some tantric ideas can be useful – especially in pregnancy.

Tantric yoga or tantric sex takes things very slowly and gently. The idea is to prolong and intensify arousal. You really concentrate on each other and what you are doing, and try to merge your sexual energy. It uses the mind to arouse as much as the body, and requires some self-control, especially on the part of any man not used to waiting to orgasm.

Synchronized deep breathing while touching is a tantric meditation. It is also something often taught in antenatal classes and can be very useful in labour. It certainly concentrates the mind and can help you 'tune in' to yourself and each other.

As for sex itself, you can alternate slow penetration and withdrawal, or try hardly moving at all. For the latter, try lying with the woman on her back with knees bent up, the man with his lower body under her legs and his upper body at nearly a right angle to her (like the 'Lying Down' position above) or any other position in which you can both lie down and be completely comfortable and relaxed. The man can insert his penis just a little way into the vagina. Then lie there hardly moving at all. There are theories about the number of minutes you should do this (e.g. around half an hour), but you do what is right for you. The idea is to relax completely and concentrate on the connection between you. If it works, after some time you should suddenly feel very aroused.

This may be well worth a try, particularly in pregnancy as it requires almost no exertion. Also, the greater blood flow to the female genitals in pregnancy and greater awareness of the area generally may help.

And More...

For more on positions and techniques, have a look at some of the sex books listed in Further Information.

Other Sexual Activity

There are of course lots of things you can do to retain physical closeness other than have intercourse or orgasm: cuddling, caressing, kissing, skin-to-skin contact, etc. Some couples enjoy describing their fantasies to each other (others wouldn't dream of it). And massage (especially full-body massage) is an excellent way of staying in touch.

Massage may be particularly appreciated by pregnant and early postnatal women who may desperately want to feel physically cared for but simply do not have the energy for making love. Relaxation is important both in pregnancy and early parenthood and it is often hard to come by. A massage can help a lot. Equally, massage allows a woman to show her love and care for her partner without involving her genitals or breasts, or any part of her body she does not feel like using. If you have not given massage before have a look at a book (see Further Information).

If one of you really wants penetrative sex or orgasm, other 'sexual' activity may be a little frustrating at times. But it is better, if you can, to overcome the frustration and keep the closeness than lose both. Make sure that you both understand whether what you are doing could lead to penetrative sex or being brought to orgasm or whether it is strictly for its own sake, with sex itself off the menu.

SEXUALLY TRANSMITTED DISEASES

If either of you has ever led a high-risk lifestyle you should ideally be checked for STDs before you try for a baby, but even if you get a diagnosis during pregnancy, most conditions can be treated or at least mitigated.

Try to go to the clinic together, and do remember not to jump to conclusions about your partner's sexual loyalty if an STD is diagnosed. It really is possible to carry some of them for many years without knowing anything about it.

Syphilis

Syphilis is the only STD routinely tested for in antenatal clinics. Some of the blood taken at an antenatal visit will be used for this test. Syphilis is extremely rare, but left untreated it can make the baby very ill. Treatment during pregnancy is easy and effective.

Chlamydia

Chlamydia is quite common. Depending on where you live, between 1 and 10 per cent of women attending antenatal clinics will have it – though many will not be aware of the fact. It is sexually transmitted but diagnosis can come many years after it was acquired. In most cases, chlamydia shows no symptoms. In women, however, it is the principal cause of ectopic pregnancy and pelvic infection and the main preventable cause of infertility.

It is possible that chlamydia may be associated with premature labour, and it can certainly damage both mother and baby. A woman with chlamydia is thought to have about a 40 per cent chance of passing it on to the baby at the time of the birth. This can give the baby sticky eye (conjunctivitis) which does not respond to the usual treatment with chloramphenicol ointment, and the baby is also at increased risk of getting pneumonia in the first six months of life.

During labour and birth (or during an abortion) infection can move up into the uterus and from there to the Fallopian tubes (through which the egg travels from ovary to uterus). This can create a generalized pelvic infection and may cause permanent infertility.

Chlamydia can be effectively treated in pregnancy with antibiotic erythromycin. The other standard treatment, tetracycline, should not be used in pregnancy as it can damage babies' teeth and bones. Both partners should be treated at the same time.

Gonorrhoea

Gonorrhoea is now rare in the UK. It is often symptomless, although it can produce a pus-like discharge and pain on urinating. It is easily treated with antibiotics of the penicillin group. Left untreated it can cause severe sticky eye in the newborn which must be treated promptly with oral penicillin.

Herpes

Most of us carry the herpes virus in some form by the time we reach our mid-twenties. It may be type 1 (cold sores) or type 2 (genital herpes) or both. For most of us herpes never causes any problems. Sometimes a woman will have her first overt attack of herpes during pregnancy. Small painful ulcers appear on the genitals, perhaps accompanied by flu-like symptoms and pain when urinating. This does not mean that she has just caught herpes. In fact it is much more likely that she has been carrying it for months or years and that pregnancy has simply precipitated the first recognizable attack.

A woman who is genuinely first infected with herpes in pregnancy and has a 'primary attack' may become very ill and is at risk of losing the baby. Fortunately this is very rare indeed. But if your partner has herpes and you do not, use a condom or abstain from genital contact from the moment you know you are pregnant.

If a woman has an active attack and is shedding the herpes virus at the time of the birth she can pass the infection on to the baby. Fortunately, despite the fact that herpes is so common, neonatal herpes (a serious illness of the newborn) is very rare. In the UK only 18 babies a year are born with it.

Some 3–5 per cent of pregnant women know they carry genital herpes. If you are one of them, you may be quoted a figure of 8 per cent likelihood of transmitting the infection to the baby. But Peter Greenhouse, Consultant in Sexual Health at Ipswich Hospital, says this is a purely theoretical figure that bears little relation to reality. In fact only 3 of the 18 babies a year born with neonatal herpes in the UK are born to women who know they have herpes. This means you have only about a 1 in 8,500 chance of your baby having neonatal herpes.

Until very recently, women who had recurrent herpes had vaginal swabs taken at regular intervals towards their due date; if the swab showed an active attack just before delivery the baby would be born by Caesarean section. Consultant Peter Greenhouse says this is no longer considered useful. By the time you know a swab is positive, he says, the woman is probably not shedding the virus any more, and if a swab is negative she may be having a new attack by the time the test results come through.

As for Caesareans, he says, unless a woman is having a visible active attack of herpes when she goes into labour they are of no value (unless there are other medical reasons). He quotes a figure that you would have to do some 100,000 Caesareans to prevent one case of neonatal herpes, in which case, the (small) risks associated with Caesareans almost certainly outweigh the benefit.

If a woman were in the midst of a visible attack when she went into labour, a Caesarean might still be done. Research trials are now going on using the anti-herpes drug Acyclovir in pregnancy. It may reduce the likelihood of transmission from mother to baby; there have been no reports so far of drug-induced damage to the baby. This treatment is, however, still in the research stage and the drug is not yet licensed for general use in pregnancy.

Warts

Most women who develop genital warts in pregnancy are doing so for the first time. This is because pregnancy provides an environment in which a wart is more likely to grow, not because the infection is new. She could have caught the wart virus at any time since she first had sex.

It is very rare indeed for warts to have any effect on the baby or on labour. They may be annoying, however, and can get worse as pregnancy progresses. The standard drug treatments, like Podophyllin, cannot be used in pregnancy. The wart can be physically removed (by freezing, cutting or possibly laser) or you can wait until after the pregnancy when it may disappear or at least get very much smaller. If the male partner gets a wart during pregnancy, use a condom while it is being treated.

Trichomonas Vaginalis

This is also rare these days. The symptoms are similar to those of Bacterial Vaginosis (BV), although the discharge is sometimes greener. There is no evidence that it presents any danger to the pregnancy or the baby, but if you are diagnosed as having it you should be checked for other sexually transmitted diseases, as should your partner. The standard treatment is with *Flagyl*, but there are restrictions on its use during pregnancy (*see page 11*).

Diseases Transmitted by Sex and Blood

(the AIDS virus)

HIV tests are available through antenatal clinics, but are not routine. You have to ask for them. Alternatively you can go to a Genito-urinary (GU) Clinic where confidentiality is guaranteed by law.

An HIV-positive mother has about a 15 per cent chance of transmitting the infection to her child, either in the womb or during the birth. The risk is higher if she has just acquired HIV and is in the acute infection stage, or if she actually has AIDS. All babies with HIV-positive mothers will be born with the antibodies and will therefore test positive, but most will have received the antibodies by passive transmission from the mother rather than because they themselves are infected.

At the time of going to press (April 1995) there is some evidence that the drug AZT given during late pregnancy may significantly reduce the chance of transmission; it is also possible that Caesarean delivery may help, though this is still uncertain. Current advice is that HIV-positive mothers should not breastfeed, as this seems to increase the likelihood of transmitting the infection. There is quite a lot of research going on in this area, so it would be as well to find out what the current medical thinking is and seek counselling before (and after) any HIV test.

Hepatitis B

Antenatal clinics can test for Hepatitis B but do not do so routinely. Hep B is transmitted in a similar way to HIV, but it has been around a lot longer and in some parts of the world it is very common. In Southeast Asia, for instance, 20 per cent of the population carries Hep B. In the UK, however, less than 1 per cent of heterosexual, non-intravenous drug users carry Hep B. If you know that you are a carrier, the baby can be vaccinated at birth and should therefore be less likely to become ill.

FURTHER INFORMATION

Books

Pregnancy and Birth

The Encyclopedia of Pregnancy and Birth, Janet Balaskas and Yehudi Gordon (Little Brown, 1994)
   (*into natural pregnancy and childbirth*)
Where to Be Born, Rona Campbell and Alison MacFarlane, National Perinatal Epidemiology Unit, (2nd edn, 1994; available by mail order only from Unit Secretary, National Perinatal Epidemiology Unit, Radcliffe Infirmary, Oxford OX2 6HE)
What to Expect When You're Expecting, Arlene Eisenberg, Heidi E. Murkoff and Sandee E. Hathaway (Simon and Schuster, 1993)
   (*very good for reference and a useful one to accompany a 'natural' approach book*)
A Guide to Effective Care in Pregnancy and Childbirth, Murray Enkin, Marc J. N. C. Keirse and Iain Chalmers (Oxford University Press, 2nd edn, 1995)
   (*summary of scientific research results on almost all aspects of maternity care – the 'bible' of research-based good practice*)
Birthrights, Sally Inch (Green Print, 1982; 1994)
   (*a parent's guide to modern childbirth; an excellent book that makes scientific research on birth available to the lay reader*)
The New Pregnancy and Childbirth, Sheila Kitzinger (Penguin, 1989)
Pregnancy Day-by-Day, Sheila Kitzinger and Vicky Bailey (Dorling Kindersley, 1990)

Becoming a Mother, Kate Mosse (Virago, 1993)
 (*a more personal guide to pregnancy, useful alongside a 'handbook'*)
The National Childbirth Trust Book of Pregnancy, Birth and Parenthood, Glynnis Tucker (ed.) (Oxford University Press, 1992)

Caesarean

The Caesarean Experience, Sarah Clement (Pandora, 1991)
Caesarean Birth in Britain: A book for health professionals and parents, Dr Colin Francome, Prof. Wendy Savage, Helen Churchill and Helen Lewison (published in association with the NCT by Middlesex University Press, 1993)

LEAFLETS
'Caesarean Birth'
'Breastfeeding after Caesarean Birth'
– available from the NCT (*see Organizations, below*)
'After a Caesarean Birth'
– to go with Postnatal Leaflet no. 3, from the Association of Chartered Physiotherapists in Obstetrics and Gynaecology (*see Organizations, below*)

Second and Subsequent

Siblings Without Rivalry, Adele Faber and Elaine Mazlish (Avon Books, 1988)
Your Second Baby, Patricia Hewitt and Wendy Rose-Neil (Thorsons, out of print)

Parenthood

The Transition to Parenthood: How the First Child Changes a Marriage, Jay Belsky and John Kelly (Vermilion, 1994)
The Beginner's Guide to Fatherhood: How to Cope with Life Before, During and After Birth, Colin Bowles (Fontana, 1992)
 (*funny and useful*)
When Partners Become Parents, Carolyn Pape Cowan and Philip A. Cowan (Basic Books, 1992)

(*report of a 10-year study; American publication which can be ordered through some British bookshops*)

The Year After Childbirth: Surviving the First Year of Motherhood, Sheila Kitzinger (Oxford University Press, 1994)
(*focuses on the mother, not the baby*)

Ourselves as Mothers, Sheila Kitzinger (Bantam, 1992)

Motherhood: What It Does to Your Mind, Jane Price (Pandora, 1991)

How Not to Be a Perfect Mother, Libby Purves (Fontana, 1986)
(*funny as well as useful*)

Goodies and Daddies: An A-Z of Fatherhood, Michael Rosen (John Murray, 1991)
(*funny and useful*)

Families and How to Survive Them, Robin Skynner and John Cleese (Mandarin, 1993)
(*a conversation between family therapist Robin Skynner and comedian and depressive John Cleese*)

Breastfeeding

The Experience of Breastfeeding, Sheila Kitzinger (Penguin, 1992)

Bestfeeding: Getting Breastfeeding Right for You, Mary Renfrew, Chloe Fisher and Suzanne Arms (Celestial Arts, 1990)
(*excellent – especially good on positioning the baby*)

The National Childbirth Trust Book of Breastfeeding, Mary Smale (Vermilion, 1992)
(*good, practical and clear*)

Sex

A Woman's Guide to Loving Sex, Tricia Barnes and Lee Rodwell (Boxtree, 1992)
(*good section on 'rekindling the flame' and very unusual in having significant sections on pregnancy and parenthood*)

Treat Yourself to Sex – A Guide to Good Loving, Paul Brown and Carolyn Faulder (Penguin, 2nd edn, 1989)

(a do-it-yourself sex therapy course, with a series of exercises – could seem daunting at first)

Sex: Why It Goes Wrong and What You Can Do About It, Martin Cole and Windy Dryden (Optima, 1993)
(simple quesion-and-answer format: everything you always wanted to know about sex but were afraid to ask – or thereabouts)

Becoming Orgasmic – A Sexual and Personal Growth Programme for Women, Julia R. Heiman and Joseph LoPiccolo (Piatkus, 1988; 1992)
(also a series of exercises, but also more general information that reads less dauntingly; parts of it of interest to those who have no trouble with orgasms as well)

Anne Hooper's Pocket Sex Guide (Dorling Kindersley, 1994)
(lots of clear pictures of positions, etc.)

Woman's Experience of Sex, Sheila Kitzinger (Penguin, 1985)

The Relate Guide to Sex in Loving Relationships, Sarah Litvinoff (Vermilion, 1992; 1993)

How to Make Love to the Same Person for the Rest of Your Life – and Still Love It, Dagmar O'Connor (Bantam, 1985; 1992)

Sexual Happiness for Women and Sexual Happiness for Men (two books), Maurice Yaffé and Elizabeth Fenwick (Dorling Kindersley, 3rd edn, 1992 and 3rd edn, 1992)
(sensible and clear: techniques and positions, and 'Problems Charts' for 'diagnosis' and solution)

Contraception
Contraception: A User's Handbook, John Guillebaud and Anne Szarewski (Oxford University Press, 1994)
The FPA Guide to Contraception, Suzie Hayman (Thorsons, 1993)

Massage

Sensual Massage: An Intimate and Practical Guide to the Art of Touch, Nitya Lacroix (Dorling Kindersley, 1989)

The Complete Book of Massage, Clare Maxwell-Hudson (Dorling Kindersley, 1988)
(*well-illustrated, clear and including a section on having a baby and massage for babies*)

Homoeopathy

N.B.
Books are useful, but it is always best to consult a qualified homoeopath if you are going to use homoeopathy to any extent.

Homeopathy for Mother and Baby, Miranda Castro (Macmillan/ Papermac, 1992)
(*pregnancy, birth and the postnatal year*)

Homeopathy for Midwives (and Pregnant Women), Dr Peter Webb (British Homoeopathic Association, 1992; 27A Devonshire Street, London W1N 1RJ; tel. (0171) 935 2163)
(*short, to the point and comprehensible to the layman; covers pregnancy, labour and the postnatal period*)

Organizations

Pregnancy and birth

National Childbirth Trust (NCT)
Alexandra House
Oldham Terrace
London W3 6NH
(0181) 992 8637
Antenatal classes, information, local postnatal groups, local activities, Valley Cushion hire

Active Birth Centre
55 Dartmouth Park Road
London NW5 1SL
(0171) 267 3006
Antenatal and postnatal exercise classes, seminars, information

Association for Improvements in Maternity Services (AIMS)
Publications:
10 Topcliffe Drive
Acklam
Middlesborough
Cleveland TS5 8HL
enquiries: (0181) 960 5585
Pressure group, information, support and advice on maternity services, including parents' rights and complaints procedures

Valley Cushion
Hire through NCT or contact manufacturers:
UT Care Products
(01709) 890655

Home Birth

NCT (*see page 195*)

Society to Support Home Confinements
Ludgate Lane
Wolsingham
Co Durham DR13 3HA
(01388) 528044
Information pack and support

International Home Birth Movement
(01734) 698275
Information pack and local contacts (worldwide)

Independent Midwives Association
Nightingale Cottage
Shamblehurst Lane
Botley
Nr Southampton
Hants SO3 2BY
(01703) 694429
Non-NHS midwives

Water Birth

Active Birth Centre (*see above*)
Information and pool hire

Splashdown Birth Pools
Pool Hire (0181) 904 0202

Caesarean

Caesarean Support Network
Yvonne Williams
55 Cooil Drive
Douglas
Isle of Man
(01624) 661269
Southern Region Co-ordinator: Linda Howes (*see VBAC below*).
Leaflets, information and support

NCT (*see above*)

VBAC (Vaginal Birth After Caesarean)
Linda Howes
8 Wren Way
Farnborough
Hampshire GU14 8SZ
(01252) 543250
*Despite its name, gives general help and information on all aspects of a
Caesarean*

Postnatal Support/Self-help Groups

Birth Crisis Network
Telephone counselling for women and men suffering after bad birth experiences (however long after!)
Write for local contact to:
10 Portrush Close
Woodley
Reading RG5 3PB

Avon Episiotomy Support Group (now national)
Lilah Beecham
PO Box 130
Weston-Super-Mare
Avon BS23 4HR
Newsletter and support network for problems with episiotomies and tears
Midlands Organizer: Gaynor Mountford, (01782) 280223
London Organizer: Sally Barrett, (0181) 482 1453

Dr Janet Menage (GP)
28 Squire's Road
Stretton on Dunsmore
Rugby CV23 9HF
(01203) 545747
Research and new support network for women suffering stress after vaginal examinations, forceps delivery, etc.

MAMA (Meet-A-Mum Association)
14 Willis Road
Croydon
Surrey CR0 2XX
(0181) 665 0357
General support network and local groups. Also specializing in postnatal depression (see below)

NCT (*see above*)
Network of local groups

Postnatal Depression

Association for Postnatal Illness
25 Jerdan Place
Fulham
London SW6 1BE
(0171) 386 0868
Information and support network (for mothers and fathers). Send SAE for information

Birth Crisis Network (*see above*)

MAMA (*see above*)
Information (including leaflets) and support network (for mothers and fathers)

Counselling

Relate (Marriage Guidance)
Look in phone book for local branch, or write to the headquarters
at:
Herbert Gray College
Little Church Street
Rugby CV21 3AP
(01788) 573241
(Some counsellors are also trained sex therapists)

London Marriage Guidance (London Relate)
76A New Cavendish Street
London W1M 7LB
(0171) 580 1087

British Association of Sexual and Marital Therapy (BASMT)
PO Box 62
Sheffield S10 3TS
Has an accreditation scheme for approved sex therapists. Also has fact-sheets on common problems

Parents' Groups/Courses

PIPPIN (Parents in Partnership/Parent Infant Network)
Mel Parr
'Derwood'
Todds Green
Stevenage
Herts SG1 2JE
(01438) 748478
Education and support programme

Exploring Parenthood
Latimer Education Centre
194 Freston Road
London W10 6TT
(0181) 960 1678
Advice, education, and counselling, and Parents Advice Line, free telephone counselling 10 a.m.–4 p.m. Mon.–Fri.

Parent Network/Parent Link
44–46 Caversham Road
London NW5 2DS
(0171) 485 8535
Education and support

GPs

Family Health Services Authority (FHSA)
See FHSA in your local telephone directory. Can give you a list of GPs in your area.

Breastfeeding

NCT (see above)
Has a nationwide network of breastfeeding counsellors

La Leche League
BM Box 3424
London WC1N 3XX
(0171) 242 1278
Information and network of counsellors

Association of Breastfeeding Mothers
Sydenham Green Health Centre
26 Holmshaw Close
London SE26 4TH
(0181) 778 4769
Information and support

Contraception

The Family Planning Association (FPA)
27–35 Mortimer Street
London W1N 7RJ
(0171) 636 7866
For leaflets send SAE; for lists of clinics and GPs offering family planning services ring or write. For immediate answers to any queries ring their information line 10 a.m.–3 p.m. weekdays on the phone number given above

Natural Family Planning Service
Catholic Marriage Advisory Council (You do not have to be either Catholic or married!)
Clitherow House
1 Blythe Mews
Blythe Road
London W14 ONW
(0171) 371 1341

Natural Family Planning Unit
Birmingham Maternity Hospital
Queen Elizabeth Medical Centre
Birmingham B15 2TG

Physiotherapy

Association of Chartered Physiotherapists in Obstetrics and
Gynaecology
Contact through the Chartered Society of Physiotherapy
14 Bedford Row
London WC1R 4ED
(0171) 242 1941

Homoeopathy

To find a homoeopath:

The British Homoeopathic Association
27A Devonshire Street
London W1N 1RJ
(0171) 935 2163
*Has lists of homoeopaths who are also trained as conventional doctors,
including their specialities (e.g. obstetrics)*

The Society of Homoeopaths
2 Artizan Road
Northampton NN1 4HU
(01604) 21400
The organization for homoeopaths who are not trained doctors

Ainsworths (*see below*)

HOMOEOPATHIC PHARMACIES (ON SITE AND MAIL ORDER):

Ainsworths
38 New Cavendish Street
London W1
(0171) 935 5330

Goulds
14 Crowndale Road
London NW1
(0171) 388 4752

INDEX